The Journey of Becoming a Mother among Women in Northern Thailand

D1602294

This publication has been supported by La Trobe University
http://www.latrobe.edu.au

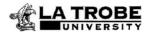

The Journey of Becoming a Mother among Women in Northern Thailand

Pranee Liamputtong

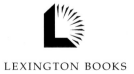

LEXINGTON BOOKS

A division of
ROWMAN & LITTLEFIELD PUBLISHERS, INC.
Lanham • Boulder • New York • Toronto • Plymouth, UK

LEXINGTON BOOKS
A division of Rowman & Littlefield Publishers, Inc.
A wholly owned subsidary of The Rowman & Littlefield Publishing Group, Inc.
4501 Forbes Boulevard, Suite 200
Lanham, MD 20706

Estover Road
Plymouth PL6 7PY
United Kingdom

British Library Cataloguing in Publication Information Available

Library of Congress Cataloging-in-Publication Data

Liamputtong, Pranee, 1955–
   The journey of becoming a mother among women in northern Thailand / Pranee
Liamputtong.
    p. ; cm.
   Includes bibliographical references and index.
   ISBN-13: 978-0-7391-2005-7 (cloth : alk. paper)
   ISBN-10: 0-7391-2005-0 (cloth : alk. paper)
   ISBN-13: 978-0-7391-2006-4 (pbk. : alk. paper)
   ISBN-10: 0-7391-2006-9 (pbk. : alk. paper)
   1. Childbirth—Social aspects—Thailand, Northern. 2. Obstetrics—Social aspects—
Thailand, Northern. 3. Motherhood—Social aspects—Thailand, Northern. 4. Infants—
Care—Thailand, Northern. I. Title.
   [DNLM: 1. Parturition—psychology—Thailand. 2. Cross-Cultural Comparison—
Thailand. 3. Infant Care—psychology—Thailand. 4. Mother-Child Relations—
Thailand. 5. Social Change—Thailand. WQ 300 L693j 2007]
RG652.L52 2007
618.2009593—dc22   2007028977

Printed in the United States of America

∞™ The paper used in this publication meets the minimum requirements of American
National Standard for Information Sciences—Permanence of Paper for Printed Library
Materials, ANSI/NISO Z39.48-1992.

To my Mother, Yindee Liamputtong,

Who becomes a Mother of eight children and raised us amidst poverty.

I love you Mum.

Without you, I would not have become who I now am.

Contents

ϰ

List of Table, Map, and Photographs

ン

Preface

 x

This book is about the journey of women becoming mothers in Northern Thailand. I wrote this book out of my own experience as a mother, as a Thai woman, and my own interest in the health and lives of Asian women. I first became pregnant nineteen years ago, and I had my second daughter four years later. My journey through motherhood was probably much like that of many mothers in contemporary societies. But, being a Thai woman living in Australia and bringing up the children single-handedly, my journey was not a silk-road one. My journey made me think about my own mother, who became pregnant ten times, gave birth to eight children, and raised us amidst poverty in Thailand. From here, I became interested in other Thai women, particularly those who came from poor backgrounds and who live in Melbourne, Australia. I undertook a research project on motherhood with Thai immigrant women and learned a great deal of the lives of women as mothers. Through this project, I realized that the social situations of the women in my study would be different from those living in Thailand. An opportunity arose when I was granted a six-month sabbatical leave by the University. That was when I commenced my research with women in Chiang Mai, Northern Thailand. I returned to Chiang Mai again in 2003, when I was given another sabbatical leave to follow up my 1999 research with Thai women. This book is born out of my fieldwork in Chiang Mai in 1999 and 2003.

Like any book, this book would not have been published without the assistance of others. In particular, I wish to express my gratitude to Katie Funk of Lexington Books who is extremely kind and supportive of my work since its conception. However, she left Lexington Books before my book was produced. Patrick Dillon and MacDuff Stewart carry the book on to the end and I am grateful to both. Like many other academics, I have to perform so many things in my working life. To write a book and try to meet the deadlines amidst other heavy responsibilities is no easy task. But I have done it, and I thank my own girls, Zoe Sanipreeya Rice and Emma Inturatana Rice for their understanding of my endless tasks. I also wish to wholeheartedly thank Rosemary Oakes who patiently read and edited the whole manuscript for me. Rosemary's assistance is deeply appreciated.

I also wish to express my sincere thanks to my colleagues at the Faculty of Nursing, Chiang Mai University, Thailand, Susanha Yimyam, Sukanya Parisanyakul, Chavee Baosoung, and Nantaporn Sansiriphun, who kindly assisted me with my fieldwork, and the Faculty of Nursing, Chiang Mai University, who generously housed me during my initial fieldwork in 1999.

The La Trobe University Publications Committee generously provided a subsidy for the publication of this book. I should like to express my thanks to the Publications Committee and La Trobe University for this support.

Parts of the book have been published elsewhere. Chapter 3 has appeared in *Sociology of Health & Illness* (27(1), 243–270, 2005); chapter 4 in *Health Care for Women International* (25(2), 454–480, 2004); chapter 5 in *Women & Health* (40(1), 79–99, 2004); and chapter 6 in *Women's Studies International Forum* (27(5–6), 589–601, 2004). Permissions from the publishers of these papers have been granted and I am grateful for their generosity.

Pranee Liamputtong
Melbourne, October 2006

Acknowledgments

ン

Chapter 3 has appeared in *Sociology of Health & Illness*

Liamputtong, P. (2005) Birth and social class: Northern Thai women's lived experiences of caesarean and vaginal birth. Sociology of Health & Illness, 27(1): 243-270. Permission is granted by Wiley-Blackwell Publishing Ltd.

Chapter 4 has appeared in *Health Care for Women International*

Liamputtong, P. (2004) Giving birth in hospital: Childbirth experiences of women in Northern Thailand. *Health Care for Women International*, 25(2), 454-480. Permission is granted by Taylor & Francis.

Chapter 5 has appeared in *Women & Health*

Liamputtong, P. (2004) *Yu duan* practices as embodying tradition, modernity and social change in Chiang Mai, Northern Thailand. *Women & Health*, 40(1), 79-99. Permission is granted by Harworth Press.

Chapter 6 in *Women's Studies International Forum*

This article was published in *Women's Studies International Forum*, 27(5-6), Liamputtong, P., Yimyam, S, Parisunyakul, S., Baosoung, C., & Sansiriphun, N., When I become a mother!: Discourses of Motherhood among Thai women in Northern Thailand, pp. 589-601. Copyright Elsevier, 2004. Permission is granted by Elsevier.

Chapter One

Introduction: Thai Women, Reproduction, and Motherhood

ใ

Maternal practices begin in love, a love which for most mothers is as intense, confusing, ambivalent, poignantly sweet as any they will experience.

(Ruddick, 1980: 344)

Motherhood—the way we perform mothering—is culturally derived. Each society has its own mythology, complete with rituals, beliefs, expectations, norms, and symbols . . . . The good mother is reinvented as each society defines her anew, in its own terms, according to its own mythology.

(Thurer, 1994: xv)

POINT OF DEPARTURE

This book is about women who become mothers in Northern Thailand. My interest in Northern Thai women stems from my own inner ambition of living in Chiang Mai, a beautiful city in the north of Thailand. I spent my childhood in the south of Thailand, but the beauty of Northern Thailand has always seduced beckoning me there. This opportunity arose when I became friends with one of the lecturers at Chiang Mai University, and through her I managed to spend my sabbatical leave in 1999 at the Faculty of Nursing, Chiang Mai University, and thus, the research project in which this book is based was born.

My first attempt to talk to the women that I am writing about was to approach my colleagues at Chiang Mai University. Here, I was hoping to be able to talk to more middle class and highly educated women. When I met her, Saijai had only one child. Saijai is from a middle class family, earned her bachelor degree from Chiang Mai University, and now lives a relatively comfortable life. Saijai had a natural childbirth, but throughout her pregnancy she made a deliberate attempt to search for "good" doctors on whom she could rely. But, this did not mean that she would follow 'all' the advice from her doctors. She read extensively books on childbirth and child care. She also sought advice from her fellow colleagues who work at the university's hospital. Her financial situation allowed her to seek the best option for her baby and herself.

It was a pleasant sunny morning in Chiang Mai when my colleagues from Chiang Mai University and I were travelling along a newly constructed highway from Chiang Mai City to Mae Chantra (fictitious name) to search for rural women who would be willing to share their lived experiences of motherhood with us. When we turned off the highway onto a narrower road which would take us to Mae Chantra, a more familiar scene of rural Thailand started to appear before us. Houses are built from cheap timber with simple designs but with more land and fruit trees, particularly *lam yai* trees (longan), around (see photograph 1). Before long, we arrived at Mae Chantra and headed for the local hospital. Here, we would meet our key person who would provide access to the local women. She greeted us and introduced us to the staff at the front desk, where many local people were waiting to see doctors and receive medication. We told them that we were interested in the local women's stories of motherhood. Everyone seemed to be impressed with this; why would we, academics from the City University, want to talk to local women about

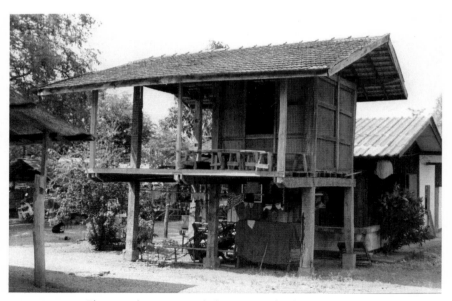

Photograph 1.   A simple house outside Chiang Mai City

pregnancy, giving birth, and rearing children when these functions are part of their everyday life? But, no one made a fuss about it; they only had smiles on their faces.

Suriya, a poor woman with two young children, was the first woman that I talked to. She elaborated on many issues, but noticeably about how difficult her life was due to poverty. She had two children in her village, as she could not afford to travel into Chiang Mai City to search for a better hospital. She was rather pale and thin. She also suffered from diabetes which, to her, had contributed to her difficult life. She was living with her parents who gave her good support. Her pregnancy was not as good as she would like because of her ill health. Due to her ill health, she would rather wish to seek help from "good" doctors in the city. But, her financial situation prohibited the granting of this wish. She did not have paid employment, but worked on the family farm. Suriya followed many of the traditional beliefs and practices that her parents told her to do. To her, this would be the way to prevent further ill health due to the childbirth process.

Saijai and Suriya represent the lived experience of being mothers in Northern Thailand. But, they are different in their social status, and as I shall show in this book, the differing social structures indeed impact how these women become mothers and the way they experience health care. In essence, each chapter will capture the lived stories of women from different social class backgrounds. And as one may expect, those who have more education, wealth, and resources will fare better in their contact with health professionals on their paths to being mothers.

STUDIES ON MOTHERHOOD AND CHILDBEARING

Although existing literature on motherhood has provided a rich understanding of motherhood and women's personal experiences of becoming 'a mother,' it has largely been examined from a Western cultural perspective. Martha McMahon (1995: 24) succinctly puts it, "motherhood is constructed as the expression of women's natural, social, and moral identity—or, rather, the identity attributable to moral women, that is married white women." Jean O'Barr and colleagues (1990) argue that motherhood reflects a culturally privileged image of white, Western nuclear family. The experiences of those who lay outside this image such as poor mothers and non-white mothers have been largely excluded. Kalwant Bhopal (1998: 485) too argues that motherhood has often been investigated from a white, Western perspective. This research often neglects "divisions based upon race and ethnicity." Current social constructions of motherhood do not reflect the realities of non-Western mothers. Hence, they are socially constructed as "other" (Bhopal, 1998: 486; Phoenix & Woollett, 1991: 18).

It is possible that women from different cultural backgrounds may have different perceptions and experiences of motherhood, as Shari Thurer (1994: xv) insightfully puts it in her writing that I present at the beginning of this chapter, and I repeat here that "the good mother is reinvented as each society defines her anew, in its own terms, according to its own mythology." In Bhopal's study (1998), for example, she shows that South Asian women living in East London see motherhood as a natural result of an arranged marriage linking to the importance of bearing male children in order to continue the ancestral line and to enhance the family pride and honour. It is through this social construction of motherhood, Bhopal (1998: 492) argues, that women are "judged as a good or a bad mother."

Motherhood contains no single meaning or a given experience. McMahon (1995) suggests that there is no universal ideal of motherhood, nor the universal experience of mothers' responsibility for their children. For some poor women, even the ideology of good motherhood dominates their self-perceptions and identities, in practice, their inadequate resources may mean that the task of motherhood is simply a struggle of trying to find food and shelter to keep their children alive. Social structures, such as class status of the women, have great impacts on the ways women become mothers and their worldly view of responsibilities toward their children.

Motherhood is complex and multi-faceted. Just as the experience of motherhood varies according to class structure and family forms (McMahon, 1995; Hays, 1996; Maushart, 1997; DiQuinzio, 1999; Lupton, 2000), culture and ethnicity also has an important effect on women's lives as mothers (Collins, 1994; Glenn, 1994; Bhopal, 1998; Liam, 1999; Feldstein, 2000). I contend that models of mothering need to take into account ethnicity and class if the voices of many women, who wish to become mothers, can be heard.

To date, the lived experiences of motherhood among Thai women are largely unknown. Earlier writings on Thai women focused on traditional childbirth beliefs and practices (see Hanks, 1963; Muecke, 1976; Mougne, 1978; Paulsen, 1984). Majorie Muecke (1984) is the only foreign scholar who has touched on status markers as mothers of Northern Thai women in more details. More recently, scholars on Thai women have concentrated their work more on different aspects of women's lives including Mary Beth Mills (1999) on women and migration, Andrea Whittaker (2000) on women's health in Northeast Thailand and her recent publication (2004) on abortion in Thailand. Both of these texts work with women from Isan—the poorest part of Thailand.

Childbearing in any society is a biological event. The birth experience is, however, socially constructed. It takes place within a cultural context and is shaped by the perceptions and practices of that culture (Lefkarites, 1992; Steinberg, 1996; Liamputtong Rice, 2000a, b). Therefore, there are many beliefs and practices relating to the childbearing process that the woman and her family must observe to ensure the health and well-being of not only herself, but also that of her newborn infant (MacCormack, 1982; Laderman, 1984, 1987; Sich, 1981; Steinberg, 1996; Jordan, 1997; Liamputtong Rice, 2000a, b). Traditional pregnancy and childbirth beliefs and practices among women of non-Western backgrounds have received much attention in the past few decades (e.g., McClain, 1975; Pillsbury, 1978; Manderson, 1981; Kay, 1982; MacCormack, 1982; Sargent, 1982; Laderman, 1987; Sich, 1981; Jeffery et al., 1988; Liamputtong Rice & Manderson, 1996; Townsend & Liamputtong Rice, 1996; Liamputtong Rice, 1999, 2000a, b).

The beliefs and practices of women in Thailand have also been documented. More than four decades ago, Jane Hanks (1963) studied childbirth rituals among women in Bang Chan village, Central Thailand. This was followed by a writing of a Thai scholar on birth customs (Anuman Rajadhon, 1987). In the last three decades, some Western researchers have conducted research relating to childbearing in Thailand including Majorie Muecke (1976) who compared Western birth with the Northern Thai way and Christine Mougne (1978) who, as part of her larger study of reproduction, examined issues related to pregnancy and childbirth in Northern Thailand. At a more recent time, Anders Poulsen (1983) examined customs and rites of pregnancy and childbirth in a northeastern Thai village. Recently, Andrea Whittaker (2000, 2002) writes about the postpartum practices of Thai women in Isan (Northeastern Thailand).

In the past several decades, rapid social, cultural, and economic transformations have changed women's lives in many parts of the world. Thailand is no exception (Muecke, 1984; Mason & Campbell, 1993; Pyne, 1994; Mills, 1999; Wongboonsin, 1995; Lerdmaleewong & Francis, 1998; Surasiengsunk et al., 1998; Yimyam et al., 1999; Lyttleton, 2000; Whittaker, 2000; Sitthi-amorn et al, 2001; Morrison, 2004). Thai women have entered the labour force as a way to increase their family income since the 1960s when the country's economy has become increasingly dependent on the global market economy (Wantana, 1982; Muecke, 1984; Mills, 1995; Yimyam et al., 1999; Lyttleton, 2000; Morrison, 2004). These changes have a profound impact on women and reproductive role (Muecke, 1984; Tantiwiramanond & Pandey, 1991; Pyne, 1994; Vichi-Vadakan, 1994; Kanchanasuk & Charoensri, 1995; Boonyoen et al., 1998; Lerdmaleewong & Francis, 1998; Yimyam et al., 1999). Malee Lerdmaleewong and Caroline Francis (1998: 29), for example, articulate that "as Thai society experiences rapid economic and social change, increased public participation by women often conflicts with their traditional roles as wife/mother, grandmother, daughter and sister. The family—considered to be one of Thailand's most important institutions—has experienced significant changes in recent years, particularly with regards to size, composition, and the role of women." Nevertheless, what it means to become pregnant, give birth, become a mother, and raise children in a changing social, cultural, and economic circumstance has largely not been given much attention in research concerning reproduction among Thai women.

This book is written with the intention to fill the gap in knowledge of cultural and social issues relating to childbearing, childrearing, and motherhood of women from non-Western societies. The focus of this book is on motherhood and reproduction of Thai women living in Northern Thailand and recounts how they perceive, achieve, maintain, and deal with their motherhood and reproduction. The book also examines how women try to adapt to changes—social, economical, and political—that affect their motherhood and reproduction. I must clearly say here that I will limit my discussions to lowland Thai women in Chiang Mai, Northern Thailand. It is impossible for me to attempt to include women from all ethnicities in this book.

WOMEN AS MOTHERS IN THAI SOCIETY

The construction of gender in Thailand does not locate neatly along rigid patterns of gender identity as understood in Western literature (Mills, 1999). Women are excluded from most highly prestigious positions of authority and leadership, but in their everyday lives, women share many responsibilities with their husbands. Mary Beth Mills (1999: 18) contends that Thai cultural practices such as equal inheritance of land, the practice of bride price and post-marital residence in the woman's home, provide Thai women with rights to access "economic and emotional resources" which are rather uncommon in many other Asian societies.

Despite a generally perceived inferior status of Thai women (Thitsa, 1980; Tantiwiramanon & Pandey 1987, 1997; Lerdmaleewong & Francis, 1998; Fongkaew, 2002), their roles as mothers and nurturers afford them a prestige and as high a status as men (Van Esterik, 1982; Keyes, 1984; Muecke, 1984; Pyne, 1994). As Christine Mougne (1978: 86) succinctly puts it, "the major role of a Northern Thai woman is as mother and housekeeper, and there is no doubt but that a woman's status is enhanced once she has borne a viable child." In the Thai society in general, and in a "female-centred" system (Potter, 1977: 20; see also Muecke, 1984; Boonchalaksi & Guest, 1994; Pyne, 1994; Morrison, 2004) observed in Northern Thailand in particular, motherhood is seen as an ability to bring a new life into the matrilineal line of the family. Girls will strengthen the matriliny of their mothers. Boys, once married, will contribute to the continuity of their wives' matrilineal line. Hnin Hnin Pyne (1994: 22) asserts that "a Thai woman's autonomy [is] bolstered by a matrilocal pattern of residence after marriage." Andrea Whittaker (2000: 70) too suggests that "female fertility is an important source of female cultural power and prestige. Through childbearing and maternity, a woman marks her status within the moral order." Pyne (1994: 22) contends "a Thai woman elevates her status and improves her inferior karma by being a responsible daughter, a reliable and supportive wife, and, most of all, a nurturing mother." Hence, being able to have children is highly valued in Thai society (Boonmongkon et al., 2001, 2002; Whittaker, 2000; Liamputtong et al., 2002, 2004). A woman is, therefore, encouraged to become pregnant as soon as possible after marriage. Recent figures show that age at first marriage among Thai women is 20.5 and age at first birth is 21.9 (Ministry of Public Health, 2002). During pregnancy, women are warned against various practices which could result in miscarriages or stillbirths. This means the survival of new babies bringing life to the family. After giving birth, the mother is well looked after by the family members so that she can rest to regain her health after a long period of pregnancy and birth (see chapter 5 in this volume). This is a reward for her for producing a child to ensure the continuity of her matrilineal line. This cultural perception makes pregnancies, birth, and the period soon after such precious events in the lives of Thai women.

Female ties among women in Northern Thailand are strong (Davis, 1974; Potter, 1977; Mougne, 1978; Muecke, 1984; Liamputtong et al., 2004). Richard Davis (1974: 9) contends that "Northern Thai social structure . . . [is] dominated by female ties." Similarly, Sulamith Potter (1977) suggests that the social structure in Chiang Mai village is female-centred with structurally significant consanguineal ties between women. For Potter (1977: 123) these strong ties are the reflections of the social structure found in Northern Thailand in "which lineality is traced through women, rather than men." Hence, significant matrilineal kin plays a major role in the way women become mothers and nurture their children. The support they receive during childbearing periods helps women to cope better with the demands of childrearing. For the whole month after giving birth, women are required to rest. All household chores including taking care of a newborn infant are undertaken by other female kin members, particularly their mothers and sisters: they are "other mothers" who provide support to mothers. Becoming pregnant and bringing a new life into the society is, therefore, perceived as strengthening female ties. It is not too surprising then that safe pregnancy and birth is most valued among the women in the Thai society. The Northern Thai women in my study are no exception.

MOTHERHOOD AS STATUS MARKERS OF
NORTHERN THAI WOMEN

Majorie Muecke (1984: 461–464) contends that women in Northern Thailand obtain "prestige" through a few means and these include "morality, the market and longevity," but most importantly motherhood. Muecke (1984: 461) suggests that "the associated resources controlled by women have been children, karma and ancestral spirits, money, and life experience." Although these resources or status markers are closely interrelated, morality and having many children are believed to be "a larger store of merit." Women in her study in Chiang Mai perceived "childbearing in the moral terms of Buddhism." As Muecke (1984: 462) puts it:

> Bearing a child improves a woman's karma both by providing a *winyan* (life principal) with a body and home for its reincarnation as a human being, and by assuring a woman's merit, when aged or deceased, through the acts of her children.

For Thai women, motherhood has long been the essence of their statuses. Nearly a century ago, Ernest Young (1907: 99) documented that "great respect [was] shown to the condition of motherhood, a wife of low rank with children being of far more importance in the family than even the chief wife, should she be childless." Infertility is seen as stigmatized among Thai people, and it can be used as a ground for legal divorce (Boonmongkon et al., 2001, 2002). It has also been the cause of many broken marriages in Northern Thailand. It is claimed that women could not live without children, although they could live without husbands (Muecke, 1984). Prior to the introduction of birth control in the 1960s, Northern Thai women controlled their fertility by having two children every three years (*saam pii song khon*). Most women continued to bear children until menopause. Hence, most Thai women would have six to seven living children on average (Knodel & Prachuabmoh, 1973). I am also one of this ideal *saam pii song khon* natural child-spacing of my mother. If a marriage is broken, children would stay with their mothers rather than with the fathers (Muecke, 1984).

Motherhood is highly valued for many reasons. As Majorie Muecke (1984: 462) puts it:

> It provided needed labor for agricultural subsistence; it provided sons who could make merit for parents by being ordained as Buddhist monks; it provided daughters to help with domestic responsibilities, to bring strong husbands into the household labor force, and to maintain the lineage through childbearing.

Children are a greater source of status for mothers than fathers. For men, Muecke (1984: 463) suggests, children are one of many different obtainable resources. But for women, almost all of women's resources depend on their children within the domestic domain. Having many children is, therefore, perceived as "a woman's wealth and her greatest resource" (Muecke, 1984: 462).

The status markers of mothers can also be clearly seen within the concept of *bun khun*. To the Thais, including Northern Thais, *bun khun* is understood as "any good thing, favour or help which is meritorious (*bun*)" (Podhisita, 1985: 39). The involvement of parents in raising children is *bun khun*. Teachers providing knowledge to students is *bun khun*, and friends helping friends is also *bun khun*. *Bun khun* is more than a duty that one must perform. The one who gives help expects no favour in return, but the beneficiary of the favour must seek opportunities to return the favour in order to express his or her gratitude.

There are two types of *bun khun*: *bun khun* by "status relation" and *bun khun* by "individual's performance" (Suvanajata, 1976). *Bun khun* by status relation is a close personal relationship and a lifelong obligation. *Bun khun* in a kinship system, particularly involving parents and elders, as well as *bun khun* of teachers are *bun khun* by status relation. For *bun khun* by individual performance, it is an interchanged relationship. One does a favour for another person and the other one feels obliged to return the favour. This circle of *bun khun* is a formal relationship. It is outside the kinship circle and has no long term obligation. *Bun khun* between superiors and subordinates, friends and neighbours are cases in point.

Bun khun obligation is highly valued and important in Thai culture. One who enters a *bun khun* relationship and recognizes it, is always admired by members of Thai society. People disapprove of and dislike whoever neglects to return the *bun khun*. One strong belief about *bun khun* among the Thai is that the debt of *bun khun* is never completely repaid. Once one falls into the circle, he/she is strongly bound by it. Additionally, *bun khun* is closely related to *bun* and *bab* (merit and demerit). This is particularly so between parents and children. One who acknowledges his/her parents' *bun khun* and repays it has gained *bun*. Thai Buddhists believe that such a person brings harmony and happiness to society. On the other hand, one who does not repay parents' *bun khun* is considered to be *khon neera khun* or *khon akatanyu* (one who does not acknowledge *khun*) and his consequence is *bab*. Neil Mulder (1985: 35), for example, sees that:

> *Neera khun*, that is, ungratefulness and not to acknowledge the moral goodness that one has received, is sin (*bab*) against the reliable order of morality and will automatically be punished by the principle of moral justice, that is karma.

Herbert Phillips's work (1965) on Thai peasant personality shows the high value of the *bun khun* relationship between parents and children. When Thai peasants were asked such questions as what they think of most when they think of their parents, they showed strong tendencies towards what Phillips calls an "obligation" toward their parents. Most of the responses were judged to show an "obligation" to a mother. Examples include: "making merit for her; her well-being; he is concerned about it; her goodness; he had fed from her breast; it was her blood that fed him; he must not forget her kindness (her *bun khun*); her *bun khun* to him; he must obey his mother" (Phillips, 1965: 157). The status of Northern Thai women, hence, can be summarized as Muecke (1984: 465) convincingly points out:

> Northern Thai women have traditionally had control as children and ancestral spirits . . . These resources demarcate the status of women as the critical earthly link in the cycle of human reincarnation. The women have been the living fulcrum between the past and the future, between ancestors and descendants, and between the dead who are to be reborn and the living who are to die.

As in many parts of the world, Thailand has become increasingly integrated into a global economy. Thai society has, thus, become more westernized and modernized (Morrison, 2004). Due to this modernization, we have seen the erosion of traditional status of Northern Thai women. There are largely two main aspects of this erosion (Muecke, 1984). Firstly, women have migrated to larger cities in search of employment and this has separated many women from the houses of their parents, from the residence of their ancestral spirits, and from their female kin. Lynn Morrison (2004: 335) similarly argues that "residence patterns in northern Thailand (and other parts) used to be strongly matrilocal, with the youngest daughter staying home and caring for the parents. Fulfilling this obligation, however, is being challenged by women who are leaving home for employment or to attend university." Secondly, fertility rates in Thailand have reduced dramatically since World War II. The development of population control policies and programs in Thailand throughout the 1960s seems to impact the reproduction of Thai women including Northern Thai. Thai women appeared to readily accept birth control. Some say that reproduction has economic implications. Urban educated women in Muecke's study (1984: 467), for example, remarked that "childbearing had become expensive; that given the new economic order, poverty was a reality or a real possibility; and that the best survival strategy for both economic and moral ends was to have fewer children than their parents had so that the children could be adequately schooled and provided for."

Others argue that the decline of fertility rates and the acceptance of birth control are markers of modernity (Mills, 1995). Things are "different today" and women perceive themselves to be taking part in this period of modernity. Morrison (2004: 339) too contends that "the Thai social economic environment is rapidly changing, and young people living in Chiang Mai are experiencing an extremely dynamic sociocultural environment," which in her study, is setting the path for dangerous sexual activities, but in my study, it is setting the path for change from tradition to modernity and this means abandoning certain aspects of Thai traditional beliefs and practices regarding reproduction and childrearing in Northern Thailand, as we shall see throughout this book.

REPRODUCTIVE HEALTH AND MATERNITY CARE IN THE THAI CONTEXT

In 2002, the population of Thailand was 62.81 million (UNICEF, 2002). In 1996, life expectancy at birth was 69.97 for males and 74.99 for females. It is expected that by 2020, male life expectancy will increase to 72.2 and female to 76.5 years (Ministry of Public Health, 2002). Females comprise more than half of the Thai population. According to the Ministry of Public Health (2002) the number of females is 31,279,000 compared to 30,848,000 males. In 2002, the fertility rate was 2.1 and the annual number of births was 1182 (thousands) (UNICEF, 2002). The Thai government has promoted the model "two child family" as part of its implementation of a major population control plan since the 1970s (Limanonda, 2000). This implementation has had a great impact on the reproduction of Thai women and the women's fertility trends in the past three decades have reflected the success of this program. In the early 1960s, the fertility rate was 6.3 but by the early 1990s, this had decreased to 2.17 (National Economic and Development Board (NESDB), 1994). According to Bhassorn Limanonda (2000: 256), the dramatic changes in Thai women's reproductive patterns are due to "the government's strong commitment to, and the effective implementation of, the population program and the active roles played by Thai women as service providers and recipients in the population control program." As much as 90 percent of family planning acceptors are women (NESDB, 1994). The most commonly used method of family planning in Thailand is female sterilization (Chintana, 1986; Whittaker, 2000).

The infant mortality rate (infant deaths per 1,000 live births) has dropped dramatically in the past thirty years; a decline from 84.3 in 1964 to 26.1 in 1996 (Ministry of Public Health, 2002). In 2002, the infant mortality rate was 25 per 1,000 live births. However, the mortality of infants under 5 years was 29 per 1,000 live births (UNICEF, 2002). Similarly, maternal mortality rate (maternal deaths per 100,000 live births) had declined significantly in the past three decades (Limanonda, 2000). In 1962, it was 374.3 per 100,000 live births (Minister of Public Health, 2002). In 2002, the maternal mortality ratio

was 44 per 100,000 live births (UNICEF, 2002). Reduction of maternal death
has been a target in Thailand's National Economic and Social Development
Plan (NESDP) as part of the development of quality of life of the Thai people. In the 7th NESDP (1992–1996), for example, the target was to reduce
maternal deaths to 30:100,000 live births at the end of the plan. At the end of
the current NESDP (1997–2001), the death rate is set to be 20:100,000 live
births (Kanshana, 1997). From the current rate, it can be seen that the Plan
has not reached its aim.

According to a report of the Safe Motherhood Project (Kanshana, 1997),
the incidence of maternal deaths in 1990 was highest in the Northern region
(45:1000.1000 live births), where this study was undertaken. This was followed by the Northeast, the South, and the Central regions respectively. By
1994, the rate had decreased significantly in every region except the South.
In 1994, the main causes of maternal deaths include antepartum and postpartum hemorrhage (39.7%) and amniotic fluid embolism (19.8%). This was followed by toxemia of pregnancy (11.3%), heart diseases (12.9%), sepsis
(8.9%), and other causes (9.5%) (Kanshana, 1997).

Antenatal care in Thailand is a health service that ideally all pregnant
women should be able to access. According to the 8th National Economic and
Social Development Plan (1997–2001), Thailand has a policy to improve the
position of women, particularly in health. As Mukda Takrudtong (1998: 3)
points out, "the Plan seeks to promote health as a way to develop the quality
of life of mothers and pregnant women by providing comprehensive reproductive health services" including the promotion of ante- and postnatal care.

According to the Ministry of Public Health (2002), all pregnant women
should have at least four antenatal care visits. However, the number of antenatal visits can be varied depending on a woman and her health-care providers.
A common recommendation will be that when a pregnant woman learns about
her pregnancy, she should visit antenatal service to register her pregnancy, re-
ferring to it as *fak thong*. The woman will attend antenatal checkups every
month before 28 weeks of gestational age, then every fortnight during 28–32
weeks and every week after 32 weeks. In 1995, 83.4 percent of pregnant
women sought antenatal care (Warakanim & Takurdton, 1998). Figures from
the Ministry of Public Health in 2001 (Ministry of Public Health, 2002), however, showed that only 76.4 percent attended antenatal care. It is difficult to
pinpoint this decrease from statistical analyses, but it clearly points to the fact
that the 7th and 8th National Plans have not been too successful nationwide.

Health care in Thailand is organized and provided by the public and private
sectors. The Ministry of Public Health is the provider of public health services. These services are also available in medical school hospitals under the
Ministry of Interior Affairs and private clinics and hospitals (Warakanim &

Takrudtong, 1998). Antenatal care is given free of charge in public health services. It is generally performed by obstetric and gynecological nurses or midwives in a normal pregnancy, but a pregnant woman may be seen by an obstetrician once during antenatal care. Obstetricians or gynecologists will be responsible for cases with high risk pregnancies (Hanvoravongchai et al., 2000). Women may, however, choose to have their own private obstetricians or gynecologists and hence have antenatal checkups in their doctors' private clinics or in the hospital where the doctor attaches himself as a medical specialist (see Riewpaiboon et al., 2005). This can be a public or private hospital. Most births, however, occur in hospitals or health-care settings.

In general, a woman will give birth where she receives her antenatal care. In the case of receiving antenatal care from a private doctor, the birth will take place in a hospital where the doctor works as a medical specialist. Antenatal care in the public sector is referred to as *fak thamada* (normal pregnancy care) and that in the private clinic as *fak piset* (special pregnancy care). Women's discourses about this care will be discussed in chapter 2 in this volume. There are costs associated with *fak piset*. The fees vary depending on the type of birth and the place of birth. In a private hospital, the fee may range from 17,000 Baht (U.S. $472—around 36 Baht per U.S. $1 at current exchange rate) for vaginal birth to 30,000 Baht (U.S. $833) for caesarean birth. Women who give birth in public hospitals need to pay an additional "gratitude fee" to the doctors who provide special care during pregnancy. These "gratitude fees" are informally set, depending on the agreement between a woman and her doctor. They are based on the Thai cultural practice of gratitude expression (*bun khun*), which can be in cash or in kind, but more so in cash (Hanvoravongchai et al., 2000; Riewpaiboon et al., 2005). This may range from 3000 to 5000 Baht (U.S. $83-$139) for vaginal delivery (Hanvoravongchai et al., 2000; Riewpaiboon et al., 2005). For a caesarean section, the fee will be much higher which can vary from 5000 to 15,000 Baht. My sister-in-law has recently given birth by a caesarean section and she paid 15,000 Baht to her doctor as a "gratitude fee."

BIOMEDICAL PRACTICES AND LOCAL KNOWLEDGE IN THE THAI CONTEXT

Western medicine was introduced into Thai society in 1923, when the Rockefeller Foundation assisted in the reorganization of the only medical school (Siriraj) in Thailand (Donaldson, 1982). The early attempts of the Foundation, according to Cohen (1989: 160), were "associated with cultural imperialism— a belief in the superiority of Western culture as manifested, in particular, in scientific medicine" (see also Brown, 1976, 1979). The expansion of Western medicine in Thai's health, illness, and health care has, however, occurred only in the 1980s (Sermsri, 1989). Due to the nation's attempt to modernize and westernize the society, childbirth in Thailand has also been corporated into the medicalization of health care (Maxwell, 1975; Muecke, 1976; Whittaker, 2000). The medicalization of childbirth, in turn, has resulted in a highly technological approach with routine hospital procedures (Muecke 1976; see also chapters 3 and 4 in this volume).

Despite the dominance of biomedicine, Whittaker (2000: 49) suggests, other non-biomedical therapies have not been totally erased. There exists other forms of knowledge which have influenced, and continue to influence, health care in Thailand (Riley, 1977; Golomb, 1985; Brun & Shumacher, 1994), including pregnancy care (Whittaker, 2000). Louis Golomb (1985: 162) contends that in most rural areas where Western health services are inaccessible or poorly equipped, local villagers continue to seek care from traditional healers similar to the way urban people would visit a general practitioner. This non-biomedical health care includes traditional healers, known as *mor boran* (ancient doctors) and medicines referred to as *ya phaen boran* (medicine derived from ancient types of practice) (see photograph 2). In pregnancy and childbirth, this also includes traditional birth attendances.

Prior to the introduction of government Western health services, care during pregnancy and birth was mediated within a family. Childbirth in Northern Thailand, according to Majorie Muecke (1976: 377), is "a thoroughly domestic event of explicit moral and social significance. The event occurs at home, in the presence of the husband, and children. Each witness has a role to play even young children might be called upon to run an urgent errand." Thai women gave birth at home and most often in the company of their husband, female kin, or traditional birth attendant (referred to as *mae jang* in Northern Thailand) (Muecke, 1976; cf. Whittaker, 2000 for *mor tamyae* in Northeast Thailand). *Mae jang* delivered births in the villages and assisted women with postpartum practices during the first month after birth. Despite the fact that childbirth in Thailand has been medicalized, in some rural parts of Northern Thailand *mae jang* still exists. Muecke (1976: 377), in her study in early 1970s, also points out that there existed two systems of childbirth in Chiang Mai: "the indigenous tradition-honoring and domestic Northern Thai system of delivery and postnatal care, and the imported medical and institutionalized Western system of obstetrics."

In accordance with the Thai Seventh National Development Plan (National Economic and Social Development Board, 1992), along with the medicalized childbirth discourse, it aimed to have 75 percent of women give birth in hospitals. This seems to be the success in Thai medicalized birth, as the majority

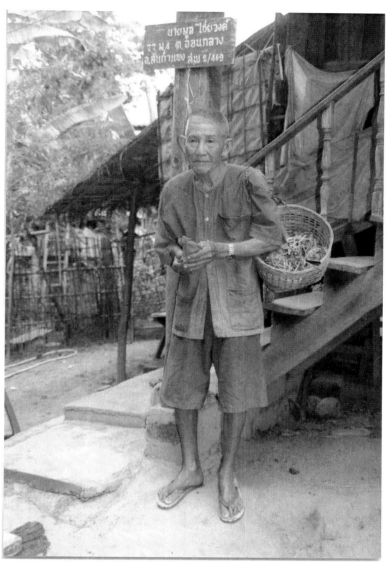

Photograph 2. A traditional healer and his herbal medicine in Chiang Mai rural area

of Thai women now give birth in hospitals (National Statistical Office, 1997; Whittaker, 2000; see chapters 3 and 4 in this volume). Of all pregnant women in 2001, 96.4 percent gave birth in health facilities, hospitals, or health centers with the assistance of Western-trained personnel including doctors and trained midwives (Ministry of Public Health, 2002). The Thai women in my study (see chapter 4 in this volume), for example, perceived hospital birth to be safer than home birth. Women articulated that there were sufficient modern medical technology and doctors who are skillful and had medical knowledge to help them if any complications occurred in childbirth. Several decades ago, Majorie Muecke (1976) and more recently Andrea Whittaker (2000) too found that Thai women in the North and Northeast adopted the Western mode of birth as they believed in the "esoteric knowledge" of the doctors, Western medications, and modern equipment used in the hospital. Natural childbirth, Whittaker (1997: 481) contends, is now replaced with "medical birth where the uterus is the centre of activity and the site of intervention by the midwife or doctor."

Despite the persistence of the traditional medical system, the rise of modern medicine in Thailand has also witnessed its destruction (Brun & Shumacher, 1994). Cohen (1989: 160) too suggests that Thai western professions assert their "dominance over other health practitioners by means of subordination or exclusion." Following Brigitte Jordan's position of authoritative knowledge (1997), Andrea Whittaker (2000: 60) contends "certain forms of knowledge based on Western, rational science have been privileged over local wisdom." In her work with women in Northeast Thailand, Whittaker (2000) points to the uneasy relationship between modern Western doctors and local villagers. By seeking care from Western hospitals, Whittaker (2000: 123) argues, "women become participants in a process wherein their bodies are constituted as sites of reform and 'modernisation' . . . This discourse seeks to rid village women of what biomedicine defines as 'superstitious beliefs' and 'traditions,' and in doing so challenges and alters the subjective meanings of female bodies and the authority of traditional knowledge." What is at stake then is the legitimacy of Western biomedical knowledge and any other forms of knowledge, particularly folk and traditional knowledge, is made subjugated in pregnancy and birth care.

THE STUDY: SOCIAL CONSTRUCTION
OF MOTHERHOOD

This book is based on my observations and in-depth interviews with thirty Thai women who are living in Chiang Mai, Northern Thailand. Fifteen women were recruited from Chiang Mai City and fifteen from the Mae Chantra sub-district, around 50 km from the municipality of Chiang Mai. This was to ensure that women from different social class backgrounds would be selected (see Nelson, 1983; Hurst & Summey, 1984). Women from Chiang Mai City were mainly from urban and middle-class backgrounds with a higher educational level, while women from the Mae Chantra sub-district were from a peasant background and had lesser educational attainment and income. The majority of the women in this study had recently given birth, but a few were pregnant when I conducted this study.

The theoretical sampling technique set out by Anselm Strauss (1987) was used to determine the required number of women. Accordingly, interviews continued until no further new data was being generated. In this study, there was little new data being generated after the thirtieth interview. The women's socio-demographic characteristics are presented in table 1.

Women in Chiang Mai City were firstly recruited through my personal network as well as through a "snow ball" sampling technique (Liamputtong & Ezzy, 2005); that is, women were asked to nominate or contact their friends or relatives who would be interested in participating in the study. Women from the Mae Chantra sub-district were first recruited with the assistance of a health worker at Mae Chantra hospital antenatal clinic. A "snow ball" sampling technique was then applied. Through these networks, all women approached agreed to participate in the study. Each woman was informed about the nature of the research and her participation. An informed consent form (in Thai) was signed once the women agreed to participate in the study. Ethical approval was sought and granted by the Ethics Committees of La Trobe University and Chiang Mai University.

The women were individually interviewed about traditional beliefs and practices regarding pregnancy and childbirth as well as background information on socio-demographic characteristics. The interviews were held in the women's homes. All interviews were conducted in Thai. Each woman was interviewed once, with the interview lasting between one to two hours, depending on the participant. The women were asked several main questions, and each was prompted with further questions to verify their explanations such as reasons for their actions/non-actions. All interviews were tape-recorded for later transcription and analysis. All interviews were transcribed in the Thai language to maintain the subtlety and meaning of the women's voices as accurately as possible. The analysis was also done from the Thai transcripts, and only those quotations which are presented in this book were translated into English. The translation retains, verbatim, what the women said, with some syntactical corrections. I translated the quotations, and these were cross-checked for accuracy by a Thai researcher who has worked with

Table 1. Socio-demographic characteristics of Thai women in this study, n=30

Age	
< 20	1
20-30	12
31-40	15
41-50	2
Religion	
Buddhist	30
Marital Status	
Married	28
Widowed	1
Living Together	1
Length of Marriage	
1-5 ys	15
6-10 ys	7
11-15 ys	5
16+	3
Education Level	
Primary	11
Secondary	7
Diploma	4
Tertiary	8
Occupation	
Home Duties	4
Self-employed	6
Government Officials	9
Farmer	3
Casual/Part-time Job	8
Number of Children	
1	14
2	14
3	1
4+	1
Family Members in the Household	
Spouse and Children	11
Spouse Children and Other Relatives	19
Family Income (in baht)	
<5,000	10
5,001-10,000	6
10,001-20,000	6
20,001-30,000	2
30,001-40,000	2
>40,001	4

me on another project. Inconsistencies between our translations were then modified to best represent the women's narratives. The study was first undertaken between January and July 1999 and a follow-up study was carried out in the first half of 2003 when I returned for some observations and discussions regarding infant care and childrearing with the women.

The in-depth data were analysed using a thematic analysis method guided by phenomenology. Phenomenology, as Carol Becker (1992: 7) argues, aims to interpret "situations in the everyday world from the viewpoint of the experiencing person." Phenomenology attempts to "determine what an experience means for the persons who have had the experience and are able to provide a comprehensive description of it" (Moustakas, 1994: 13). In this study, the interview transcripts were used to interpret how women described their meanings and experiences of motherhood in their everyday lives. Their responses were then organised into coherent themes, as presented in each chapter. The focus of my analytic approach was on identifying not only themes and patterns that the women recounted about their lived experience (Liamputtong & Ezzy, 2005), but also "contradictions, ambivalence and paradoxes" of their narratives (Lupton, 2000: 53). Women's discourses concerning their childbearing and childrearing experiences are presented and their names have been changed for confidentiality. My interpretation of the data relies heavily on women's accounts given in the in-depth interviews. Due to time constraints, I could not employ other means such as intensive participant observations for data collection. Hence, I cannot claim a triangulation of information generated.

Chiang Mai, where this study was undertaken, is the second largest city in Thailand, with about 200,000 people (Morrison, 2004; World Facts Index, 2004). It is situated in the northern part of Thailand (See map 1). Historically, Chiang Mai was known as the capital of the Lanna Kingdom or the Million Rice Fields Kingdom, which is now Northern Thailand. Chiang Mai was founded by King Mangrai in 1296 and was an independent kingdom until 1932 when it became a province of Siam, a former name of the present day Kingdom of Thailand. Chiang Mai has its own distinct social and cultural heritages. People refer to themselves as *khon muang* who originated from mixed ethnicities including *Lawa*, *Mon*, and *Tai Yuan*. Chiang Mai people speak a Northern Thai dialect known as *kham muang*. *Kham muang* has its own vocabulary and tones, hence, the Northern Thai language may not be understood by those from Central Thailand (http://www.chiangmai1.com/chiang_mai/history_3.shtml).

Among major cities in Thailand, Chiang Mai is markedly caught in the social, cultural, and economic transformations. Lynn Morrison (2004: 329) points out that "catering to Western tourists, by definition, entails exposure to, and familiarity with, Western social behaviour. Changes, whether they are in the forms of food, music, or clothing styles, are pervasive and widely accepted, and

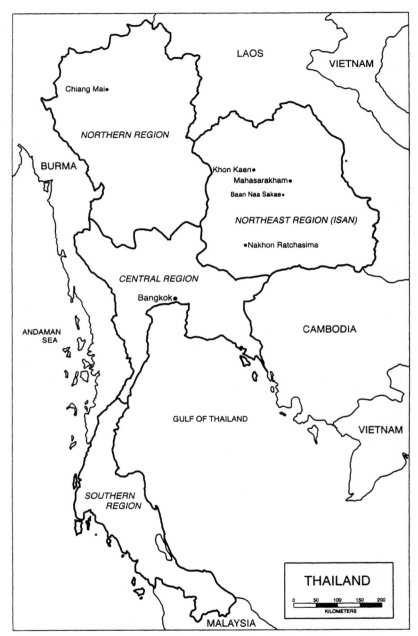

Map 1.   Map of Thailand

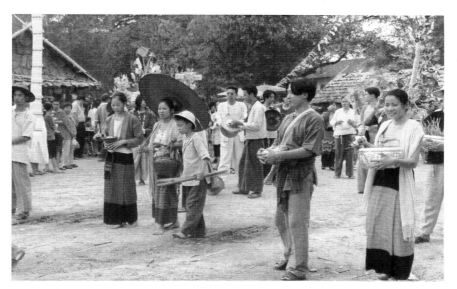

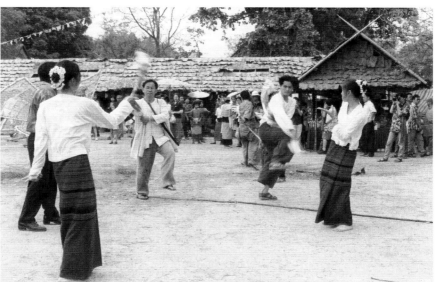

Photographs 3 & 4. Traditional costumes of Chiang Mai people during the Thai New Year in April

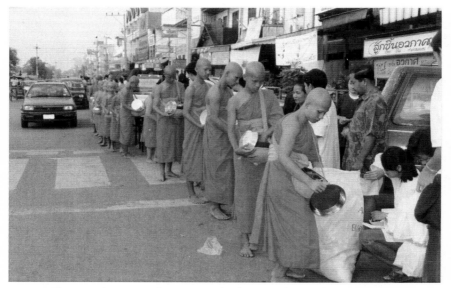

Photograph 5.   Monks receiving food at a market in Chiang Mai town

they have had an enormous impact on young people." Chiang Mai, "traditionally a predominantly rural and agrarian society," is "now marked by increasing
urbanisation, one effect of which is the increasing mobility of women. Wide-
spread industrialization is attracting young women and men from rural areas to
cities like Chiang Mai for employment and education. The migration of young
people to cities has led to the erosion of the extended family as the unit of authority" (Morrison, 2004: 329).

   As in many major parts of Thailand, the construction of modern roads and
a new fast highway has made transportation more accessible and easier than
before. For a trip from many villages to the city of Chiang Mai, it now takes
about half an hour. Therefore, people from the villages prefer to commute to
work in the city where employment with regular incomes can be sought
(Fongkaew, 2002). This is applicable to the preference to seek health and maternity care in the city by rural women who can afford this expense.

ABOUT THIS BOOK

This chapter begins with a general overview of motherhood and childbearing
and childrearing from a cross-cultural perspective. Evidence from empirical
research regarding childbearing and motherhood is discussed in relation to
the intersections of class, gender, and ethnicity. An overview of Thai women

as mothers in the north of Thailand is discussed in the chapter. I have also introduced the research on which this book is based.

Chapter 2 discusses antenatal care and the experience of pregnancy among the women in my study. In this chapter, I address the issue of authoritative knowledge in antenatal care among Thai women in Northern Thailand. Women assert that their doctors know best about their pregnancy and what they should or should not do. They follow medical advice, most often, without any question. Women wish to make sure that they do everything right to ensure the safety of the birth and a healthy child. Some middle-class women wish to have choices and control over their pregnancies and the antenatal care they receive by choosing their own doctors. These opportunities are denied to rural poor women due to their financial hardships. Medical advice to rural poor women does not seem to take into account the social circumstances of the women. Most poor women are unable to follow dietary advice from their doctors. In this chapter, I come to a conclusion that to many Thai women, the cultural authority of biomedicine pervades. Despite several decades of campaigns for reproductive choices among women's movements, these notions are still problematic in Thai antenatal care.

Chapter 3 contributes to a sociological understanding of women's childbirth discourses. I will show that the lived experiences of birth differ between individual women. Social resources such as financial resources and education play a salient role in shaping the embodied experience of birth among women in Northern Thailand. Due to their "everyday lifestyle," middle-class women have more control over the experience of childbirth than that of the rural poor women. The middle-class women are able to choose where to give birth, have access to private care, and actively seek medical technology as a way to have control over their births. Their material resources enable their choices. These choices seem to be denied to the rural poor women. But, not all rural poor women are passive victims of their material resources. No matter how little the resources women have, they use them. Hence, there are some poor women who actively seek birthing care that enables them to have more control. But, regardless of their social positions (urban middle-class or rural poor), obstetric interventions are commonly experienced, and most women perceive caesarean birth in a positive light. Several discourses are employed to explain these findings including women's interpretations of their lived world including risk and the medicalization of childbirth in Thailand. Taking a feminist standpoint, I argue that differences between women need to be taken into account in providing care to women in childbirth so that sensitive and appropriate birthing care for women can be achieved.

In chapter 4, I examine how Thai women perceive and experience childbirth in hospitals. The women's narratives reveal that childbirth was managed within the medical system. The women believed that safety was the primary reason for their choice of birth in a hospital. Women's embodied experiences with hospital birth reveals the "passivity" discourse; women accord total trust to their doctors and very rarely question the many routine procedures in hospitals. It seems that in Northern Thai hospitals the involvement of women's partners or their "significant others" is kept to a minimum. Of interest among postpartum care provided in Thai hospitals in the North is the use of a spotlight to help heal the episiotomy wound. This is an adaptation of Thai traditional confinement practices in the era of modernity. The use of a spotlight in hospital not only provides the women with symbolic ritual but is believed to assist them in the healing process. Women in general were satisfied with postpartum care received during their hospital stay, except for rooming-in practice. The data suggest some differences between rural poor and urban middle-class women in terms of hospitals of birth, the opportunity to have a family member at birth and so on. Again, it is clear that middle-class, educated women are able to exercise their choices and control over their childbirth experiences much more than rural poor women. I argue that care provided to women during birth needs to take into account women's emotional and subjective experience so that sensitive birthing care can be achieved. This will make childbirth of many women a more positive experience

Chapter 5 examines the traditional postpartum beliefs and practices which still exist in Northern Thailand today. Beliefs and practices remain an essential part for postpartum care for women in Northern Thailand and have important consequences for women's health and well-being. Many Thai women see their reproductive health problems as the consequence of inadequate postpartum practices. Thai women also believe that the effects of postpartum taboos would continue for the rest of their lives. Although the traditional postpartum beliefs and practices abound, the level of adherence differs according to the social structure of the women and their families. Poor rural women seem to hold on to their traditions more strongly than their urban counterparts. Urban middle-class women in particular embody modernity in their thinking and behaviour concerning postpartum practices. But, modernization has brought with it medical dominance. Due to their medical knowledge, doctors retain authority over both knowledge and status. The consequence of this dominance is the attempt to dismiss local traditional knowledge and practices. Although the pattern of traditional postpartum beliefs and practices is changing, it is still observed in Northern Thailand. I contend that postpartum care for women incorporates local traditions so that women's health can be optimized at the time when they are in the most vulnerable stage of their lives.

The discourses of motherhood among Thai women from Northern Thailand are discussed in chapter 6. Motherhood has several meanings among Thai women in this study. Common to all women is the perception that motherhood is not an easy task. Some women believe that motherhood means self-sacrifice and endless concern, for others motherhood brings joy and pleasure to their lives. Women also mention that becoming a mother makes them appreciate the love and sacrifice which their mothers have had for them. This perception is linked with the Thai cultural concept of *bun khun* (gratitude). Some women believe the processes of being a mother depletes their health. Low satisfaction with motherhood and its consequent unhappiness found in several studies with women from Western societies does not exist in this study. This may be due to the expectations of motherhood in Thai society as well as support the women receive from their families when they become mothers. Women are different in their meanings and experiences of motherhood. These differences, I suggest, must be recognized so that a clearer understanding of motherhood can be achieved. Only then can health services and care be made more meaningful to many women who have decided to become a mother.

In chapter 7, I examine infant feeding practices among the women in my study. Infant feeding practices are indeed contentious issues. The findings suggest that "infant feeding is a moral minefield." The ways that women can be judged or judge themselves is clearly articulated in this study. Infant feeding decisions are not only about nutrition, but more importantly, are about morality. Whether the women intend to breast or formula feed, they attempt to construct "an image of themselves as moral members of society." Mothers' intention to breastfeed is culturally constructed as an act of a good mother. These women follow the rules knowingly, and hence, were not questioned about their maternal morality or felt the need to justify their intentions. Breastfeeding could be perceived as "evidence of being a good mother who is not only knowledgeable but who is also prepared to act on that knowledge." But, this also holds true for mothers who intend to bottle-feed despite some societal ambivalence about their infant feeding intentions.

The discourse on breastfeeding amongst the Thai women in my study relates to ideals of motherhood. Most often, women refer breast milk to "mother's milk" (*nom mae*). This emphasizes the mother and child relationship ideal. The belief that it is a mothers' blood that creates her breast milk and the characteristics of a mother is transferred to her child through breast milk reinforces the interconnection between a mother and her child. It is clear that both breast- and bottle-feeding mothers see themselves as "knowledgeable rather than ignorant." I suggest that we must be mindful that women do not necessarily lack knowledge to make decisions about infant feeding, but that "there are other significant factors at play." And in this study, I have shown that there are other significant factors including work and insufficient milk dictate whether women choose to breast- or bottle-feed their infants.

Finally, in chapter 8, I discuss the cultural construction of childrearing and infant care in Northern Thai society. I show that Thai mothers observe and practise many socially and culturally acceptable tasks to ensure the health and well-being of their infants. Mothers see themselves as responsible parents, and hence, follow numerous rules to avoid risks which may pose threats to the health and well-being of their infants. This attempt, I claim, is used as a means to prove that they are good and moral mothers.

I conclude the chapter with a postscript to show that becoming mothers is no easy task for the women in this study. All women, poor or better off, have to travel through a long journey of childbirth to taking care of their newborn infants. As in any society, childbearing and childrearing and infant care perceptions and practices are constantly subject to social, cultural, political, and economic changes. How the Thai mothers may deal with these changes remains to be seen.

Chapter Two

My Doctor Knows Best:
Antenatal Care and
Authoritative Knowledge

Ж

Whenever the doctor made the appointment for me I would go. If I missed it, and if the baby was born abnormally, the doctor would not take care of us. The doctor said at the beginning that if I missed the appointment, he would not be responsible if anything happened. So, I was afraid and just went all the times.

(Srinang, a rural poor woman)

INTRODUCTION

The concept of "authoritative knowledge" has been a focus of discussion among medical anthropologists who engage in the critical analysis of the social production of knowledge (Kaufert & O'Neil, 1993; Lindenbaum & Lock, 1993; Rapp, 1993). These writers have focused their attention on "the privileged status of biomedicine as a realm of knowledge, which is separate from other cultural or social domains and which is seen as objectively valid" (Sargent & Bascope, 1996: 214; see also Rhodes, 1990; Lock & Scheper-Hughes, 1990). Discussion of authoritative knowledge in childbirth was initiated by Brigitte Jordan, and since her first publication in 1978, there have been several researchers applying this concept in different childbirth domains (See Davis-Floyd, 1992; Lazarus, 1994; Davis-Floyd & Sargent, 1997; Whittaker, 2000; Root & Browner, 2001).

Brigitte Jordan (1997: 56) convincingly argues that in any social situation, there exist different kinds of knowledge, but some kinds of knowledge may have more weight than others. And this becomes known as "authoritative knowledge" (Jordan, 1993, 1997). The reason for this, as Jordan (1997: 56) argues, may be due to its "efficacy" because it may "explain the state of the world better for the purpose at hand." It may also be due to "structural superiority"; that is, it is associated with a stronger power base. Under most circumstances, however, it is usually both. Drawing on Jordan's concept of "authoritative knowledge" (1997, 1993), I examine the experience of antenatal care of Thai women in Northern Thailand in this chapter.

All too often, in order to legitimize one kind of knowledge as authoritative, other kinds of knowledge are either dismissed or devalued (Armstrong, 1983; Jordan, 1993, 1997; Lupton, 1995; Turner, 1995; Whittaker, 2000). Alternative knowledge such as embodied or folk knowledge may be "correct," but regarded as "backward, ignorant, naïve, or simply trouble makers" (Jordan, 1997: 56; see also Ehrenreich & English, 1978). Therefore, this alternative knowledge does not "count." As Jordan (1997: 58) succinctly puts, "the power of authoritative knowledge is not that it is correct but that it counts." As I shall show in this chapter, very often women possess embodied knowledge about the stage of their pregnancy but this knowledge is dismissed as naïve. Only knowledge gained from pregnancy tests would "count" as legitimate. As well, folk knowledge relating to safe pregnancy and childbirth has been subscribed by women, it has been subjugated as backward and ignorant within the domain of Western biomedicine (Cohen, 1989). As we have seen in the Thai society, traditional midwives and other healers have been subjugated and do not hold similar privileged status as those from biomedical backgrounds (Cohen, 1989; Whittaker, 2000). Folk knowledge similarly does not count.

According to Michel Foucault, power relations are "produced and reproduced through the everyday activities and social encounters" (Lupton & Fenwick, 2001: 1012; see also Foucault, 1980; Armstrong, 1997; Lupton, 1997; Turner, 1997). Jordan (1997: 56) too sees authoritative knowledge as constructing through "an ongoing social process that both builds and reflects power relationships within a community of practice." Eventually, she argues, all those involved in the process learn to "see the current social order as a natural order, i.e., as the way things (obviously) are." Through this social process, the patients come to see the knowledge of medical professionals as authoritative.

In clinical encounters, authoritative knowledge is constructed through unequal power relationships between the medical professionals and the patients (see Ehrenreich & English, 1978; Porter & Macintyre, 1984; Rapp, 1993; Browner & Press, 1996; Lupton, 1995, 1996, 1997; Georges, 1997). As implied in Foucault's genealogies of power/knowledge (Foucault, 1980) that "power is possessed by . . . a class, a people and power is centralized in the law, the economy and the State" (Sawicki, 1991: 52), those who possess more knowledge also possess more power and in many cases, as in the medical domain, I argue that they also possess authority. While Jordan (1997: 58) indicates that she does not consider authoritative knowledge as "the knowledge of people in authority positions," in this chapter, I follow the argument put forward by Carolyn Sargent and Grace Bascope (1996: 214), who suggest that authoritative knowledge indeed "reflects the distribution of power within a social group." By this, I mean the power between the doctors and the pregnant women. In Sargent and Bascope's study (1996: 232), they show that "the social status and cultural authority of biomedicine created through discourse and embedded in the status of physicians maintained its ideological dominance." To Andrea Whittaker (2000: 124), authoritative knowledge "involves differential power relations between differing knowledge systems and different groups in society." Hence, authoritative knowledge is seen as what Pierre Bourdieu (1977) refers to as "cultural capital"; knowledge that is distributed unevenly among different social classes in a society, and this knowledge allows the holders to possess the status of dominance. Almost all Western-trained doctors in Thailand are those from higher social status with more wealth, education, and power. As I shall show, to our women, doctors' authoritative knowledge incorporates their authorities as well. My position in this chapter, hence, departs from Jordan's theoretical background at this particular point.

Childbearing in any society, as I have suggested in chapter 1, is a biological event, but the birth experience is also socially constructed. It takes place in a cultural context and is shaped by the views and practices of that culture. Therefore, there exist numerous beliefs and practices relating to the childbirth process that the woman and her family must adhere to in order to ensure the health and well-being of not only herself, but also that of her newborn infant (MacCormack, 1982; Laderman, 1987; Jordan, 1993; Steinberg, 1996; Liamputtong Rice, 2000a, b, c). Taking Jordan's argument (1997), if folk or cultural knowledge is constructed through a consensus of "what is thinkable and unthinkable" (Georges, 1997: 91–92), folk knowledge, I argue, can then be construed as authoritative knowledge in the context of my study. Folk knowledge has been incorporated into the lives of Thai people and in childbirth in the forms of traditional beliefs and practices. In childbirth, women are instructed to follow dietary and behavioral regimes to ensure safe pregnancy and childbirth (Mougne, 1978; Muecke, 1976; Liamputtong Rice, 2000a, b; Whittaker, 2000). In this chapter, I shall show that women regard some folk knowledge as authoritative, and they would incorporate this knowledge into their pregnancy care. However, in some cases, folk knowledge may clash with biomedical knowledge, and it may mean that folk knowledge has to be surrendered.

Since authoritative knowledge is consensually constructed, it is, therefore, persuasive. Authoritative knowledge then has the possibility of "powerful sanctions." Individuals may be able to move between different forms of knowledge (see Root & Browner, 2001), but in certain boundaries and at certain times, they may have to surrender to knowledge of those in authority. In situations of structural inequality, such as in clinical care, often medical knowledge gains authority and hence sanctions and devalues and de-legitimizes others in doing so (Browner & Press, 1996: 1420). It also often "serves as grounds for action" (Sargent & Bascope, 1996: 213). I shall show in this chapter that, in antenatal care, women posses embodied knowledge and may wish to follow folk knowledge, but they may eventually give in to sanctions and authoritative knowledge of their medical professions, making them adhere to biomedical care of pregnancy.

In antenatal care, as in childbirth, there is evidence that women tend to accept medical knowledge as legitimate. In Brigitte Jordan and Susan Irwin's study (1989: 20), they found that "most women willingly submit themselves to the authority of the medical view" and the women believe that their physicians act "in their own . . . best interests." Maureen Porter and Sally Macintyre (1984) too show that women in Aberdeen see doctor's advice as legitimate, as they believe what the doctor recommends has been well thought out and, therefore, it must be the best option for them. Although there are women in Robin Root and Carole Browner's recent study (2001: 208) who resist antenatal norms, those who comply have strong faith in the authoritative knowledge of their medical professionals. These women consult and seek advice from their doctors regarding diet and behaviors. The women not only "privilege biomedical know-how," but also "relegate the non-bio-medical to the realm of non-credible."

How does this phenomenon come about? Ellen Lazarus (1994: 27–28) argues that in many parts of the world, childbirth has been seen as a medical event and controlled by the medical professions. This medicalized view sees childbirth as "potentially pathology" and that "something can go wrong at anytime." This has put women under the control of the medical professions. As Lazarus (1994: 27) succinctly puts, if women do not do "everything" like following the advice of doctors, it is their responsibility if the mothers do not have a "perfect" birth, or a healthy baby, and they must be blamed for it. This is a powerful message that pregnant women receive. It is not too surprising then that women come to believe that their doctors know best about their childbirth, and they have to rely on medical knowledge to ensure that they have done everything possible to ensure a healthy birth (Lazarus, 1994).

In this chapter, I examine the extent to which authoritative knowledge is prevalent among women in Northern Thailand. Specifically, I look at what middle-class and rural poor women have to say about their antenatal care and the extent to which they adhere to the hegemony of Western medical discourse and whether women, within the Thai context, have choices or control over their pregnancy.

PREGNANCY AND EMBODIED KNOWLEDGE

Embodied knowledge, according to Carole Browner and Nancy Press (1996: 142), is referred to as "subjective knowledge derived from a woman's perception of her body and its natural processes as these change throughout a pregnancy's course." Accordingly, women possess knowledge about the changes in their bodies, and they often are able to diagnose their pregnancies long before other means may confirm it (Jordan, 1997; Davis-Floyd, 1992; Martin, 1992). This embodied knowledge is equalized to the concept of "haptic" in Root and Browner's recent writing (2001: 201). Women adopted "haptic" including "emotions, fatigue and hunger" as a means to acquire and access knowledge of their pregnant bodies during the early months in their pregnancies. Similar to women throughout history and cultures, women in my study used their embodied knowledge to diagnose their own pregnant state. Though not all women subscribed to this, the most common of all was that they missed their period and that they started to notice a change in their bodily parts, particularly the enlargement or soreness of their breasts. Some noticed their bodily weight as they became thinner and the loss of their appetite as a phenomenological indicator of pregnancy.

Despite their embodied knowledge, some urban and educated women wished to be sure about their pregnancy by having a pregnancy test, as Patanee, an urban woman, remarked:

> I wanted to have a child and had been waiting for it, so as soon as I felt that it must be, I had a pregnancy test to see if I really became pregnant. And, it was positive.

It is important to note that to all women, including the women who learned about their pregnancy from a pregnancy test kit (a technological means), their embodied knowledge was not sufficient enough for them to be certain about their pregnancy. All women wished to have their pregnancy confirmed by a medical professional, most often a doctor at a local hospital or an obstetrician at a private clinic. The women's attempts clearly point to their trust in the knowledge of their medical professionals. Sira, an urban woman, said:

> My breasts become bigger and my menses came late, so I went to buy a pregnancy test from a pharmacy shop to test if I was pregnant. It was positive so I went straight to a hospital to have my pregnancy confirmed.

ANTENATAL CARE AND
AUTHORITATIVE KNOWLEDGE

As soon as their pregnancy was confirmed, all women sought antenatal care (*fak thong*). Women who were older who believed they were more "at risk" due to their advanced age and women with a first pregnancy were particularly eager to do so. Women believed that having put themselves under those who have authoritative knowledge such as their doctors, they could at least avoid any negative situations that might arise during pregnancy (see also Root & Browner, 2001). Siriporn, an urban well-educated woman, explained: "I *fak piset* (had special care) with a private obstetrician for both of my pregnancies. As soon as I knew I was pregnant I went to *fak thong* [register for antenatal care]. I was an older woman and I knew that I might be at risk."

All attended antenatal checkups throughout their pregnancy. It is noted that none of the women, both rural and urban, ever missed any antenatal appointment. They all made particular efforts to attend their appointments. Malai, a rural woman, said she never missed any antenatal checkup, as she was afraid that the doctor would be angry at her if she did, and hence, she did not dare to miss any appointment. The experience of Srinang, a rural woman who had her antenatal care in a public hospital in Chiang Mai City as I have given at the beginning of this chapter, clearly showed authoritative knowledge of a medical profession.

Some women kept the appointment on schedule due to their concerns about their doctor's medical knowledge. This is what Warunee, an urban educated woman, remarked:

> I never missed the appointment. I tried to make sure that the doctor would see me on time. I felt considerate as I had *fak piset* with him and he did not really charge me that much, so I went according to the appointment. Also, I did not want to see that any problem happened. Say for example, the appointment was on the 10th, but I went on the 14th, the doctor's prognosis/diagnosis would be wrong. I was worried about that, so I went on the time we had made.

Other women said that they were more concerned about the health and well-being of their fetus. By having a regular checkup, the doctor's knowledge would help them to look after their pregnancy better.

> I never missed an appointment . . . because I was afraid if there was anything wrong with the baby. Sometimes, I couldn't feel the baby movement in my abdomen. Because I am a new mother, I often could not feel it, so I panicked. So, when it was a time to go for a checkup I would go and talk with the doctor about my concerns . . . I went every month. (Pimpilai, an urban woman)

Kesara, a rural uneducated woman, too remarked that:

I never missed an appointment. I was there exactly whenever the doctor had made the appointment for my baby. It would be good for the baby because if I let the doctor check it, then I would know if the baby is healthy or not.

A vaginal examination, a common practice in many countries, was also carried out in the Thai antenatal care. But, not all women were subjected to a vaginal examination. For those who underwent the examination, they expressed their fears and said they could feel the pain when the doctor was performing and also afterwards. Despite this, women were happy to "go along" with the flow and follow their doctor's authoritative knowledge, as Warunee, an urban woman, said:

> I had a vaginal examination . . . The doctor wanted to do it, so I gave him my consent. I thought it was a normal way of medical care, it was the way that doctors do for a pregnant woman. So, it should not be any bad consequences and so I agreed.

The gender of a doctor seems not to be an issue among the women who went through a vaginal examination. In the mind of many women, all doctors, males or females, possess medical knowledge, and hence, they have authority to perform a vaginal examination, and as patients, they should not feel too concerned about it. Malai, a rural woman, explained when she was asked about her concern:

> When the doctor did the vaginal examination, I did not really feel anything. I did not feel shy or ashamed even though the doctor was a male doctor. He is a doctor, so I should not feel shy about it. When he wanted to do, it I just went along with it.

Authoritative knowledge of a doctor was more obvious among women who had prior negative pregnancy outcomes (cf. Root & Browner, 2001). This was true for both the rural poor and urban educated women in my study. Somehow, these women believed that because they did not follow medical or folk knowledge strictly enough that the pregnancy went wrong. Ruchira, a rural woman, miscarried with her previous pregnancy. With her present baby, she would welcome whatever the doctor told her to do. She had a vaginal examination so that the baby would be safe. She said:

> The doctor did a vaginal examination on me but I did not feel shy because I wanted my baby to be safe. I lost my first one through a miscarriage so I wanted the doctor to take care of me with this pregnancy.

Wilai, a middle-class and well-educated woman from Chiang Mai City, also lost her first child through a stillbirth. Due to this, she too subjected herself to medical knowledge. She attended all antenatal checkups. She also requested and insisted on having all prenatal tests including ultrasound and chorionic villus sampling (CVS) to ensure the well-being of her baby, despite the fact that her private obstetrician did not recommend any. Due to her persistence and also her advanced age, eventually her doctor ordered three ultrasounds and performed CVS.

> After I had CVS, I felt good about it because I had a test to ensure me that the chromosomes were normal. I felt that I had done the best for this baby because I lost the last one.

By putting themselves under the authoritative knowledge of their doctors, women felt that they had done the right thing. When Saijai, an urban middle-class woman, was asked how she felt when a doctor was performing an antenatal checkup, she said:

> I felt happy when the doctor told me that the baby was strong and healthy. So, when the doctor was doing a checkup I felt good inside myself.

THE CULTURE OF ANTENATAL CARE: *FAK PISET* OR *FAK THAMADA*

Most women from Chiang Mai City in my study had a special care (*fak piset*) with their obstetricians or gynecologists. These women were mainly from a middle-class background, well-educated, employed in a secure employment, and had a secure financial situation (cf. Riewpaiboon et al., 2005). Those from Mae Chantra district, except for a few women, tended to have a general antenatal care (*fak thamada*). They were poor and had a lower level of education. Most of them worked their farms or stayed at home. Financial constraints were common among these women. As there were costs associated with *fak piset* including medical consultation fees and the cost of transportation, poor women did not have the same access to *fak piset* as did the women in the city. In my study, twenty women received antenatal care from private obstetricians or gynecologists, and the majority of them were women from Chiang Mai City. Ten women received care from nurses or midwives and sometimes local doctors at local health centers, and most of them were from Mae Chantra district. Kesara, a rural woman from Mae Chantra district, said she had antenatal checkups with local health personnel at her local health station (center) and she only saw any doctor or midwife who was on duty. Similarly, Srinang, a rural woman also from Mae Chantra, only had her antenatal care at a public hospital in Chiang

Mai City. She said: "I went to have antenatal care as a public patient where most poor women go. I didn't have *fak piset* or anything. I saw any doctor according to my turn." This is the opposite of Sinjai, an urban middle-class woman, who had her antenatal checkup with her obstetrician/gynecologist at his clinic or at the hospital when he was on duty. For Sinjai, a continuity of care was then ensured throughout her pregnancy.

The well-being of their fetus seems to be the central concern of women who chose *fak piset* as a means of antenatal care. To a degree, the women in my study believed that by adhering strictly to antenatal care and the advice of their doctors, their fetuses would be healthy and safe, and in some ways, might even prevent undesirable pregnancy outcomes such as physical and mental abnormalities in the fetuses. Patanee, an urban well-educated woman, contended that she had *fak piset* with her private obstetricians, as she was worried about the health and well-being of her fetus.

> At the beginning, I was so worried and afraid; would the baby be normal or not! I was so worried because I have seen crippled children and I felt so pity for them. I thought if they were my children, it would be difficult for the children and it would be a long time burden for parents too . . . So I wanted special care from my private doctor and never missed the appointment.

For some women, issues of choices and controls become apparent. There were a few middle-class women who would actively seek doctors whom they could trust to take care of them during pregnancy. Pimpilai, an urban educated woman, elaborated:

> My menses were late, so I went to buy a pregnancy test to make sure that I was pregnant. Then I asked my aunt whom should I go to see, as this is my first pregnancy and I did not know a good doctor. My aunt recommended Dr [X] as he has a very reputable work history . . . He has a good reputation of taking care of a mother and a baby. So, I felt relieved that I could trust someone who would take good care of me.

Warunee, an educated woman from Chiang Mai City, said she selected her own doctor if he or she could match with what she wanted. This is what she said:

> I chose this doctor because I know him, but I did seek information about him prior to going to see him. I would look for the doctor's reputations, such as this doctor prefers a natural birth and wants a woman to help herself more, or that doctor likes giving a woman a caesarean and likes blocking woman's back or not, and so on. After all the information about these doctors, I chose my own.

Sinjai, an urban woman, had difficulty with conceiving. Hence, she actively sought information about a gynecologist who could help her. Through a brother of her husband, she learned that there was a new doctor who had just graduated from the USA and had a good reputation in assisting women to conceive. In her case, she believed that a good doctor would enable her to have children.

> It was necessary for me to have a good doctor because this doctor would advise me about the safety of the fetus. He would have to control my weight and constantly provide me with medication and so on. And he was very good, indeed.

PRENATAL SCREENING AND DIAGNOSTIC TEST AND DOCTORS' RECOMMENDATIONS

Women were also recommended by their doctors to undergo prenatal screening such as ultrasound to screen for any abnormality or check the progress of the fetus. But, this recommendation was not given by all doctors. Some doctors did not recommend this even though they provided a special care (*fak piset*) to a woman. It appears that doctors, in at least the northern part of Thailand, are not all prepared to use medical technology. Sirin's doctor did not recommend her to have an ultrasound, as:

> The doctor said it was not really necessary. Also it was expensive to have this test too. He said it was not necessary because the baby was healthy and strong and he usually did a routine antenatal checkup anyhow. (Sirin, an urban middle-class woman)

Pimpilai, an urban middle-class woman, did not have an ultrasound either. She said her doctor did not recommend it. However, it was also her own concern about the safety of the fetus that she did not ask the doctor to recommend one.

> My doctor did not tell me to have it, and I did not want to have it either. I could have a girl or a boy, this did not matter. From what I have heard, why should we subject our baby to any tests. Why should we interfere with the baby who is lying peacefully in our womb? . . . I think this was my first pregnancy and I should not have any problem, and my doctor did not recommend it. I was only 28 then and very healthy. I didn't have any problem with my pregnancy either. So, I did not have one.

For those doctors who advised the women to have an ultrasound, in the minds of the women, there were good reasons for it. Saijai, an urban woman for example, said that her doctor organized three ultrasound scans for her because she had a frequent abdominal pain. The doctor wanted to make sure about the condition of the fetus; hence, ultrasounds were organized. Kesara, a rural woman, had an ultrasound when she was five months pregnant, as she became pregnant soon after she had a vaccination for German measles. She told us:

> The doctor wanted to make sure that my baby is normal because of the vaccine I had prior to my pregnancy. The doctor told me not to become pregnant soon after the vaccine, but I did. So, he gave me an ultrasound just to check if the baby is okay.

Siriporn, an urban middle-class woman, was over 36 when she became pregnant for the first time. She was classified as an "at risk" mother. Hence, her doctor recommended an amniocentesis test.

> The doctor said he would like me to undergo an Amnio because I was over 35. However, he also said that it was up to me, but he would like me to do it. So, I did go along.

Siriporn also had an ultrasound when she was four months pregnant due to a sudden bleeding. The doctor thought she might miscarry, so an ultrasound was organized. Fortunately, her cervix was not totally opened. And so, he ordered her to have a total rest, and the baby was safe.

Prapaporn, an urban woman, had an ultrasound when she was five months pregnant. Her doctor advised that the fetus seemed to be too big, and he was concerned that she might have a twin pregnancy. Prapaporn said she was worried about undergoing an ultrasound, as she thought it might be dangerous. However, her doctor used his authoritative knowledge to reassure her that he only wanted to "have a good look" at her pregnancy. So, she agreed.

Pimpan, a rural woman from the Mae Chantra district, had her second child after 35 and her doctor wanted her to have amniocentesis as she was in the "at risk" group (over 35). She agreed as he recommended. However, at the local hospital there was no facility for the doctor to do a test, so it was arranged for her to travel into the town. When she turned up at the town hospital, the doctor did not do the test, but just conducted a routine antenatal checkup. She was puzzled about the change, but did not question. She told us:

> Because the doctor thought it was all right for me not to have it, then it should be ok. He did a regular checkup on my pregnancy, so I thought it should be ok too. I trust my doctor.

AUTHORITATIVE KNOWLEDGE AND
INSTRUCTIONS DURING PREGNANCY

Authoritative knowledge of medical professionals became very clear when women talked about their diet and behaviors during pregnancy.

Diet during Pregnancy

According to tradition, women are advised to be cautious about certain food-stuffs during pregnancy (cf. Wilson, 1973; Weise, 1976; Snow & Johnson, 1978; Laderman, 1984; Nichter & Nichter, 1996; Liamputtong Rice, 2000a, b; Whittaker, 2000). Most often, women are warned to avoid any foodstuff re-ferring to as *khong salaeng* (allergic foodstuff) (see Liamputtong Rice, 1988). Thai people take *khong salaeng* seriously, as it is said that the consumption of *khong salaeng* can cause health problems and perhaps death in the moth-ers. During pregnancy, *khong salaeng* may have a negative impact on the health and well-being of a fetus. In the context of pregnancy, *khong salaeng* include pickled and fermented food such as pickled cabbage, spicy hot food, bamboo shoots, egg plants, and anchovies. Women are told to consume only half of a banana, as eating a whole banana may result in a birth obstruction. Consuming shellfish and Northern Thai relishes during pregnancy will pre-vent the perineum from drying out properly after giving birth. Similarly, the consumption of Thai eggplant during pregnancy will cause anal pain after giving birth or during a confinement period.

But, very often when asked if there is anything they should eat or should avoid during pregnancy so that the baby will be strong and healthy, women would first refer to the authoritative knowledge and advice of their doctors as a way to follow rather then tradition. Pimpilai, an urban woman, told us that:

> My doctor kept telling me that I should not eat too much, that I should eat good food, like milk and fruit, so that I would not have digestion problem, and that I should avoid tea, coffee and soft drinks. If I felt like a soft drink, he said I could have some but not too much.

Saijai, an urban middle-class woman, similarly explained:

> When I saw my doctor, he would ask me how many cups of milk I drank per day. I said just one, and he would ask me to take two cups, one in the morning and one in the afternoon . . . I don't really like milk because I always feel that I will vomit after drinking it, but I tried my best to drink some milk as the doctor told me to do.

Prapaporn, another urban middle-class woman who followed her doctor's advice strictly, said:

> I mainly ate according to my doctor's advice. I asked my doctor if I needed to take any extra medication, but the doctor said I was healthy so I did not need any medication to nourish my body, only eat good and right food and never miss any antenatal checkup. This would be substantial to ensure my pregnancy.

Medical advice about diet during pregnancy was taken very seriously by women who had experienced a miscarriage or those who desperately needed to have children. This is what Ruchira, a rural poor woman who lost her previous child through a miscarriage, said:

> I must drink milk and eat good food so that my body and the baby would be strong. When I was pregnant I would eat according to my doctor's advice. I would not touch a soft drink, cigarette, or alcohol as the doctor told me because I desperately wanted to have children.

Authoritative knowledge and doctor's advice regarding diet was somewhat problematic for poor women. As most doctors recommended drinking milk and consuming good food as a means to improve the health of their fetus, it was difficult for poor women due to their financial constraints. Srinang, a poor woman from Mae Chantra, had this to say:

> Women living in my situation [being poor] would not be able to afford too much good food during pregnancy. We could only eat according to our meager means. At most, we can afford some milk. But, to eat like women in the city do, it is impossible for us.

Traditionally, Thai women may consume some traditional medicines to ensure the health of their fetus and prepare for an easy birth. One common herb used by Thai women in the North is *pu loai* or *plai*—a ginger-like plant. Traditionally, its root is boiled with water and this is consumed by a pregnant woman. However, most women in the study did not wish to take any herbal medicine during pregnancy due to their fear of harming their fetus. But, they would take whatever their doctor prescribed them.

> I never used traditional medicines during my pregnancy, but took only what the doctor prescribed for me. We should not use a traditional medicine because it may have a harmful affect on the baby. We should use only medicines recommended by our doctor; just take whatever the doctor advises. (Ruchira, a rural woman)

Behaviors during Pregnancy

Tradition dictates that pregnant women must take many precautions for the safety and well-being of their fetuses. These include avoidance of rigorous activities and sexual intercourse. Traditionally, pregnant women are cautioned to avoid intercourse as the activity is believed to cause a miscarriage in early pregnancy and stillbirth in late pregnancy. However, women sought advice from their doctor if they should have sex during pregnancy. Pimpilai, an urban educated woman, elaborated:

> My doctor advised that we could have sex during pregnancy but he said it should not be too vigorous. He said we should not have it in the first one to three months, as the fetus is in the process of getting attached to the womb. Having sexual intercourse may disconnect the fetus from our womb [a miscarriage]. But, after four months we can have sex, but not too vigorous as the fetus may be affected [miscarry] . . . Also, the doctor said that if we have sex, we may pass on some diseases to the baby. So, my husband was afraid and he stopped having sex since I was seven months pregnant.

In the mind of Kesara, a rural woman, if there was no danger in having sex during early and late pregnancy, why should the doctor tell them not to have sex during these periods. Siriporn, an urban woman, too said that she did not have sex during her pregnancy although her doctor said that it was all right in the middle trimester. She and her husband understood that the doctor's advice must have some good reasons, and so they decided to have total abstinence during pregnancy.

Wilai, an urban educated woman who lost her first child through a stillbirth, was very cautious about sexual intercourse during pregnancy. She sought advice from her obstetrician and was told that it was all right to have sex only in the middle trimester.

> I consulted my doctor if we should have sex, and he advised me that we could have some but he also advised what to do to ensure that the baby would not miscarry. He said we could have some, not to avoid it at all.

Although women tended to follow their doctor's advice, in some situations they might not. Ruchira, a rural woman, said her doctor advised her to take some exercise during pregnancy. However, due to her history of a miscarriage, she did not do so, as she feared that she might miscarry again. It seems that women only follow authoritative knowledge if it makes sense to them and does not threaten the well-being of their fetus.

AUTHORITATIVE KNOWLEDGE
AND FOLK KNOWLEDGE

As in other parts of Thailand (Golomb, 1985; Jirojwong, 1996; Whittaker, 2000), other forms of knowledge continue to influence pregnancy care of women in the North. Pregnant women in the North are given advice by their mothers or people of older generations about the preparation derived from Northern Thai folk knowledge for the birth of their baby. One notable cultural belief and practice which almost all women mentioned was the advice to consume *pak plang*; a vine-like green vegetable which is believed to make women give birth easily (see photograph 6).

The vegetable is rather slippery in its texture. Being "easy slipped" symbolically indicates having an easy birth. However, women believed that the vegetable would make the baby's body slippery, hence facilitating an easy birth. Some said that they consumed this vegetable throughout their pregnancy but others mentioned that it is only taken toward the end of their pregnancy. The vegetable can be prepared in a soup form with chicken meat or stir-fried with pork mince.

> I ate a lot of *pak plang* during pregnancy. *Pak plang* is a soft vegetable and we make into hot soup, a Northern style hot soup . . . We eat all the leaves and the water because it is slippery and this makes the baby slip out easily. (Isara, a rural woman)

Also a common practice is to gather *pak plang* and *maiyarab* plant (another vine-like green plant) and make them into a loop and then boil them with water. A pregnant woman then showers with this herbal water. When she is taking a shower, the loop will be put on her head. This is believed to facilitate an easy birth. Women who were told to do so had no problem in following this cultural practice, as it did not interfere with their pregnancy or harm their fetus.

Another common advice given to pregnant women was to drink *nam maprow*—fresh juice from a young coconut. It is believed that if a mother drinks fresh coconut juice during pregnancy, the baby is born without fatty stuff on its body and scalp, hence, the baby will look clean and beautiful. This belief seems to be pervasive regardless of the woman's social background. Pimpilai, a woman from Chiang Mai City, explained:

> Older people tell me to drink fresh coconut juice from seven months onward. They say when the baby is born its scalp will have no fatty stuff and it is clean. They say fresh coconut juice is pure. My husband would buy me fresh coconut juice . . . Ironically, the baby was still born with fatty stuff anyhow, even though

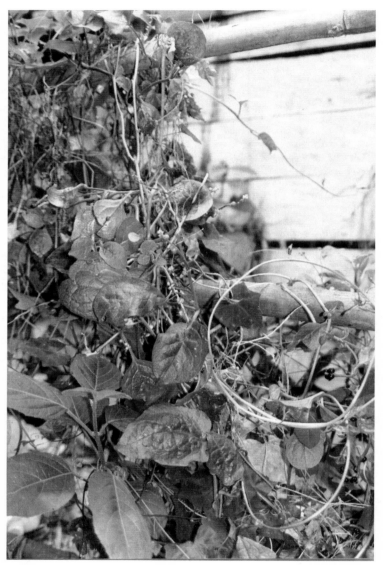

Photograph 6:   Pak Plang

it was not too much. However, I followed what older people told me for their sake. They have more experiences than me, so I wanted to follow their advice. My husband would buy me one coconut each day and I would drink it.

To buy a fresh coconut each day throughout pregnancy seems to be feasible for women who are financially sound. For some, particularly poor women, this became difficult and in some cases impossible. Malai, a poor woman from Mae Chantra, said that she believed that drinking fresh coconut juice would make her baby beautiful at birth, but she could not afford to drink it too often.

> I only had fresh coconut juice on and off; did not have it throughout pregnancy because I did not have enough money to buy them. One coconut costs me 10 baht and my husband had to go into town to buy it. We could not really afford it.

Women were also told to keep doing light exercises such as walking or doing light household chores throughout pregnancy to facilitate easy birth. As this cultural practice seems to coincide with their daily life, most women had no difficulty in following the advice.

> Most often people would tell me to do some light work and walk. They say do not just sleep or lie down all the time. If you do some work it will be easy to give birth. I walked a lot during pregnancy. (Pimpilai, an urban woman)

However, any rigorous or heavy work is not advisable during pregnancy, as this can lead to a miscarriage. Most women were cautioned about this and tried to avoid rigorous activities. But, for some women, particularly poor women, this would be difficult for them to follow or even impossible. Malai, a rural poor woman, remarked:

> People told me not to lift heavy things because they said the baby would be harmed. But, I still had to do it. We work in a farm and I often have to lift an engine to draw water into the farm. Even when I was eight months pregnant, I still had to help my husband doing that.

Isara, another rural poor woman, also commented on the difficulty in observing this cultural knowledge. She remarked:

> My parents told me that I should not do too much heavy work and that I should rest more . . . so that I won't miscarry . . . But, talking about women in our situation [being poor], not to work hard or not to work at all is impossible. We have to continue working throughout pregnancy for survival.

Another strong cultural knowledge that women were cautious about during pregnancy was not to prepare anything including nappies and clothes for their baby. Advance preparation would result in the death of the unborn baby. As Saijai, an urban woman, explained:

> I did not prepare anything for my baby. It is a taboo in this region. They say if you prepare anything for your baby, you won't get the baby [meaning the baby will die]. The baby will not have a chance to be born, so people would tell me not to prepare anything.

When asked what she did with things that the baby needed, she said:

> Well people would buy things for you before you gave birth, but they would keep them until they were sure that the baby was born and the baby was safe, then they would bring them to you. Also, my mother would prepare most things for me and she would bring them into the hospital for me.

Most rural poor women in this study tended to follow cultural beliefs and practices, as they believed in the wisdom and knowledge of older generations. Pimjai, a rural woman from Mae Chantra, did not prepare anything for her newborn baby.

> If you are talking about a northern Thai cultural practice, we cannot prepare anything in advance. People believe that something will happen to the baby if we prepare things for it. The baby will be in danger [die]. I did not prepare anything for my baby. When older people tell you anything, you need to believe them and follow their advice. They know better, and it is not good for us if we do not follow their advice.

However, folk knowledge was seen to be less relevant to their pregnancy among urban women in Chiang Mai City. Women stated that they had become more modernized than their older generations. Tradition and modernity is a dichotomy of being in the old days and new times (Mills, 1999). Andrea Whittaker (2000: 5) suggests that this dichotomy is captured in the way that Thai people at all levels refer to "perceived differences" between past and the present. For Mary Beth Mills (1999: 13), modernity points to "a break between past and present as distinctive ways of life, contrasting the achievements and forward-looking potential of modern life against the failings or disadvantages of backward-looking 'tradition.'" The tradition/modern dichotomy is also a perceived disparity between "the status and prestige of images and practices" between the urban middle and upper classes and rural communities. According to Whittaker (2000: 5), this dichotomy is best seen as disparity "in the distribution of wealth and power as matters of having (or lack of) knowledge and experience of 'modern' ways rather than as inequalities of class."

Being modern, in the mind of some women, meant an abandonment of traditional knowledge. Araya, an urban woman, for example remarked that she did not follow any folk knowledge regarding safe pregnancy given by her mother, as this knowledge belongs to the old day (*samai khon*). A modern person (*khon samai may*) need not observe the traditions belonging to old beliefs. Similarly, when asked about traditional beliefs and practices concerning a preparation for an easy birth in the North, Pimpilai, an urban woman, answered that she no longer believed in traditional knowledge.

> I don't know about it because I am a modern person. I don't really believe in the old way. This does not mean that I look down on traditional beliefs and practices, but I don't really hear about them either, so I don't know much about them. Now, whatever a woman does in pregnancy is not relevant, as if she has a difficult birth, she just has to go into hospital and she has an operation [caesarean].

Often, women received two sources of authoritative knowledge: medical and folk. Lakana, a woman from Mae Chantra district, said her doctor advised her to drink a lot of milk, to eat food containing the five food groups and not to consume pickled food or smoke or drink alcohol. Her mother, however, told her to observe traditional food such as consuming *pak plang* for an easy birth and take only half a banana so that she could avoid an obstructed birth. Isara, a rural woman, provided a logical explanation of why she followed any authoritative knowledge:

> I followed what other people told me to do because I wanted to make sure that the baby would be fine. I was afraid that the baby would be abnormal. If I didn't follow their advice, and if something was wrong with the baby, it would be difficult for me as a mother and it would be difficult for the crippled baby. If the baby was abnormal, then I had to find money to cure him and that would be difficult for me. The baby would also be looked down on by others in society because a crippled person is not valued in the society.

More often, women could incorporate both systems without difficulty. But occasionally, folk knowledge clashed with medical knowledge. Pimpilai, an urban woman, talked about her experience of diet during pregnancy:

> People of older generations would always tell me to eat for my baby too, but Dr X would say it was not necessary. He said I didn't have to eat for my baby. He said what I ate would go to the baby, so I didn't have to eat two serves because I would put too much weight on.

In some cases, women chose to only observe medical knowledge rather than traditional knowledge. Sinjai, an educated woman in Chiang Mai City, said about her diet during pregnancy that:

> People advised me to take Chinese herbs or Thai traditional medicines . . . so that the baby would be strong and clever, but I did not believe in it. I mainly consumed good food like milk, egg and other food stuffs which provide all sorts of good things rather than taking Chinese herbs or Thai herbs, as I was afraid that these would be dangerous to my baby.

CONCLUDING DISCUSSION

Brigitte Jordan (1993, 1997) and Michel Foucault's insights (1973, 1980) into the unequal power relationships between those who possess medical knowledge (such as medical professionals) and those who lack it (such as pregnant women) are particularly apparent in this study. The women in my study perceive that medical professionals have authority and legitimate authoritative knowledge. As Jordan (1993, 1997) notices, in certain situations, such as in antenatal care, some forms of knowledge count and others do not, regardless of "truth value." This is clearly mirrored in this study. Although women suspected that they became pregnant and even though they sought a pregnancy test to confirm it, they would still seek confirmation from medical professionals. Women come to trust authoritative knowledge more than their own embodied knowledge. In the minds of these women, authoritative knowledge seems to "count" more than their own "bodily experience." But, for some women, their embodied knowledge encourages them to follow authoritative knowledge. As illustrated in Carole Browner and Nancy Press's study (1996), women who have experienced a miscarriage, for example, would eagerly incorporate medical advice into their everyday lives. This is, for these women, the way to ensure a safe pregnancy and the well-being of their fetuses. This can also be clearly seen in the women's narratives in Robin Root and Carole Browner's study (2001). The women who complied with authoritative knowledge expressed their ideas that their miscarriages were caused by not following the advice of their doctors. The women in my study, who have prior adverse pregnancy outcomes too, eagerly do so for the well-being and safe journey of their fetuses.

The medicalization of childbirth in Thailand health care, like childbirth in many Western societies, makes medical knowledge "supersede" other kinds of relevant sources of knowledge such as the woman's prior experience and the knowledge she has of the state of her body (see Ehrenreich & English, 1978; Duden, 1993; Root & Browner, 2001). The woman herself comes to believe that the professional's medical knowledge is the best for her (Jordan, 1997: 61). It seems, as Maureen Porter and Sally Macintyre (1984) have pointed out in their study of antenatal care in Aberdeen, women see that whatever is recommended by their doctor must be "best" for them.

Jordan's assumption that authoritative knowledge is more pervasive when it is related to technology (1997) is not contested in the Thai context (at least in this study). As Eugenia Georges (1997: 92) points out, most kinds of technologies have authoritative power due to their "symbolic (and practical) value" and "their association with experts." Carole Browner and Nancy Press (1996: 141) point out in their study that few U.S. women refused the offer of ultrasound or other forms of antenatal diagnostic screening. This is because the women see "information derived from technology as inherently authoritative knowledge" (see Davis-Floyd, 1992, 1994; Rapp, 1987, 1999). Some urban women in my study too seek a pregnancy test kit to confirm their embodied knowledge, and they willingly accept prenatal screening and diagnostic tests recommended by their doctors. However, not all women and medical professions in Northern Thailand totally succumb to medical technology.

I find that the class background of the women determines the extent to what women can do as well as their wishes to follow medical advice during pregnancy (see also Martin, 1992; David-Floyd, 1994; Lazarus, 1994; Zadoroznyj, 1999). Only those who have better education and employment are in a better position to seek a special care from their own medical professionals. Unlike their urban middle-class counterparts, to rural poor women access to special care is denied and they have to rely on public health care. To these women, issues of choice are not an option for them. As a public patient, they only receive care from a doctor who is on duty. Poor women are, therefore, as Ellen Lazarus (1994: 26) puts, "constrained by the conditions under which they have babies and the kind of care open to them."

Despite the fact that rural poor women do not have as good access to good care as those urban middle-class women, it is noted that the acceptance of authoritative knowledge is more prevalent among these women than urban women. What can account for this? Authoritative knowledge is derived from the power structure of the medical profession. As Lazarus (1988: 45) argues, "the control of medical knowledge, [and] technical procedures . . . creates a world of power for the medical profession." The lack of medical knowledge does not enable women of any background to challenge power/knowledge of their doctors or other health-care providers. With little or no education, rural poor women are further pushed under medical dominance. Power structure can clearly be seen from the fact that women fear offending their health-care providers, particularly their doctors, as they may not be helped if anything happens. And this may explain why they do not miss any appointment made for them. Rural poor women are even more cautious about this, even though they have to travel a long distance to see their doctors. To offend their doctors is unthinkable.

But, I also notice that although some rural poor women accepted authoritative knowledge of their doctors, in reality many recommendations could not be easily incorporated into their everyday lives. A recommendation of taking "good food" such as milk, for example, was impractical and unrealistic to many poor women due to their financial constraints. It is too costly for them. Medical advice is all too often offered without sufficient regard of the realities of women's lives (Browner & Press, 1996: 150; Root & Browner, 2001).

Similarly, although folk knowledge tended to be observed by rural poor women, to follow this may pose some difficulties for some of the women. To drink a fresh coconut each day throughout pregnancy, for example, seems to be feasible for women who are financially sound. But, particularly for poor women, this becomes difficult and in some cases impossible. In addition, any rigorous or heavy work is not advisable during pregnancy as this may cause a miscarriage. For poor women, this caution may be difficult to heed if at all, as they still have to perform their heavy routines throughout pregnancy.

Although folk knowledge has been utilized by women and men alike in Northern Thailand (and other parts), it has become structurally inferior to Western biomedicine (Lee, 1982; Golomb, 1985; Cohen, 1989; Sermsri, 1989; Brun & Shumacher 1994). Folk knowledge is largely and gradually losing its authoritative status in the urban Thai context. This is because birth in urban Thailand, as in many other parts of the world, has been medicalized and this has placed pregnant women under medical authoritative knowledge. But even so, folk knowledge is still prevalent among those in rural and remote areas where modern medicine has not totally penetrated. As I have shown, some women in this study still observe Thai traditional practices during pregnancy. Rural poor women in particular adhere more to their folk knowledge than urban middle-class women. The practices are passed on by those who possess traditional knowledge. Although there is evidence in other contexts that folk and medical knowledge can coexist and complement each other (Golomb, 1985; Sermsri, 1989; Whittaker 2000; Liamputtong Rice, 2000a), within the context of this study, women can only follow folk knowledge which is not sanctioned by, or clashes with, medical knowledge. In certain circumstances, women have to surrender to the authoritative knowledge of their doctors.

According to the Foucauldian perspective, power relationships often fluctuate and are not always one-way (Foucault, 1980; Lupton & Fenwick, 2001; Root & Browner, 2001). I do see some middle-class women in this study, although they are in the minority, wanting to have some control over their pregnancy and having an active say in their antenatal care. They do seek the authoritative knowledge of the medical professionals, but they also make sure that they have their own choices regarding from which they should seek care. They actively gained knowledge about a "good doctor" on whom they could rely. Such women are able to challenge the power of their doctor by asserting that they are not a passive patient but a knowledgeable consumer. But, as Lazarus (1994: 29) points out, "taking control of one's life and body is a middle-class perspective." In this study, the women's class, education, and financial positions enable them to do so. This is denied to those rural poor women, who are restricted by limited knowledge and overwhelmed with economic problems. Hence, they have limited choices and control over their pregnancy (cf. Whittaker, 2000 in her writing about poor women in Northeastern Thailand).

My findings have implications for quality antenatal care and further research in Thailand. First, women from different social class backgrounds may receive different clinical services. The possible consequence of *fak piset*, for example, is that it may discriminate against quality of antenatal care of those who cannot afford such special care, those who have to conform to *fak thamada*. This culture of antenatal care practices, hence, may create a two-tiered system where urban middle-class women receive better quality of care including the choices of perceived "good" doctors and continuity of care, and rural poor women can only access a second-class care (cf. Riewpaiboon et al., 2005). This reinforces inequality among social classes in health care.

Second, my findings show that authoritative knowledge is less likely to be detrimental, but rather, it does not take into account the social positions of women and their living circumstances (cf. Root & Browner, 2001). It may be more appropriate if a doctor spends time discussing with the women their needs and constraints prior to giving any advice so that his or her recommendations to the pregnant woman may be more pragmatic. And third, my findings apply mainly to authoritative knowledge of medical professionals, particularly obstetricians and gynecologists, in antenatal care. As nurses and midwives also play a major role in the provision of antenatal care in Thailand, it may be important to examine the role of authoritative knowledge of a nurse or midwife or other health personnel dealing with pregnancies so that sensitive and appropriate antenatal care may be achieved. Unfortunately, it is beyond my capacity to discuss this issue in this study.

In conclusion, in the minds of many Thai women in this study, the cultural authority of biomedicine pervades. My data clearly show that the construction of "legitimate health knowledge" (Abel et al., 2001: 1145) has resulted in the marginalization of other kinds of knowledge including embodied experience and cultural knowledge. And, if medical hegemony continues to be constructed through the social process of unequal power relationships between those who possess knowledge and those who lack it, authoritative knowledge continues to be the discursive practice that shapes the lived experience of many pregnant women. This will make an attempt to improve the cultural relevance and sensitive care amidst the mainstream of dominant culture of Western medicine and medicalization a challenging task indeed.

Chapter Three

Birth and Social Class:
Vaginal or Caesarean Birth?

ϰ

I thought a lot about choosing caesarean because I was worried about the well-being of my baby. If I had a big body, I might try to experience child-birth pain as most mothers have to go through. I wanted to know what it would be like to experience pain in childbirth. But, I was afraid that I might lose the baby through childbirth process, so I decided to have a caesarean instead of vaginal birth. My doctor said if he was me he would try a vagi-nal birth, and if things did not go well then I could have caesarean. But, I did not wish to try to risk my baby's life, as I have lost one already.

(Wilai, an urban educated woman)

INTRODUCTION

Childbirth, as I have suggested in the previous chapter, is a significant human experience, but its social meaning is shaped by the society in which birthing women live. Childbirth and its management, therefore, occur within the so-cial context of the event (Romalis, 1981; Lefkarites, 1992; Liamputtong Rice & Manderson, 1996). Childbirth in most modernized societies, according to Maria Zadoroznyj (1999: 267), has become "emblematic of the phenomenon of medicalisation," as many medical interventions are utilized to monitor and control the woman's body. Ellen Lazarus (1994: 25) too argues that birthing care, "with its reliance on technology, is both a forceful practice and a pow-erful ideology." This ideology has markedly influenced pregnant women's perceptions and management of their birth. To many women, birth is no longer seen as a natural event, but an event to be managed using technologi-cal interventions.

Of these prevalent medical interventions, caesarean birth is the most common. Caesarean sections have increased in developed countries undergoing modernization (Barros et al., 1996; De Muylder, 1993; Sakala, 1993; Campero et al., 1998; Castro et al., 1998; Cai et al., 1998; Belizan et al., 1999; Hopkins, 2000; Tatar et al., 2000; Wu, 2000; Leung et al., 2001). Thailand is no exception. Caesarean section rates in Thailand have increased from 15.19 percent in 1990 to 22.44 percent in 1996. In 1996 alone, rates of over 59 percent occurred in private hospitals (Hanvoravongchai et al., 2000). Caesarean section rates also differed according to region. In the capital city, Bangkok, where the majority of women are from upper- and middle-class backgrounds, the rate was nearly twice that in Northeast Region, the poorest region of the country. Of interest too is that Ministry of Public Health (MOPH) provincial hospitals were responsible for 32 percent of total national caesarean births in 1996 (Hanvoravongchai et al., 2000). These hospitals are located in the main provincial city where most private doctors practice. Hence, childbirth in Thailand has become medicalized and professional delivery is being promoted. However, there is little data documenting the perceptions and experiences of birth of Thai women in a medical environment. In this chapter, I examine lived experiences of caesarean and vaginal birth among the Northern Thai women in my study.

This chapter contributes to a sociological understanding of women's childbirth discourses in three ways. First, my discussion draws on a qualitative approach that explores women's lived experiences of childbirth. As such, I examine the discourses upon which the women draw when making sense of their embodied experiences and interpretations of childbirth, whether vaginal or caesarean. Second, the chapter attempts to move our understanding of women's experiences and practices of birth away from the biomedical discourse that permeates medicalized birth in Thailand and elsewhere. Last, I situate my interpretations in the social context within which the birth occurs. As such, I attempt to look at differences and similarities between women from rural poor and urban middle-class backgrounds.

SOCIAL CLASS, CHOICE, CONTROL, AND CHILDBIRTH

It is well established, sociologically, that attitudes, expectations, and access to health care differ according to the individuals' social structures. Mildred Blaxter (1990), for example, points out in her analysis on "fatalism/activism" in health behaviors that these concepts are socially structured along class lines. Middle-class individuals tend to be more activist in their orientations and practice, and hence, have more sense of control than working-class individuals, who tend to be much more fatalistic. Alan Blair (1993: 40-41) too, demonstrates differing personal control of distress and illness along class lines. Working-class participants "gave less value to personal control." They tended to say that recovery from illness (such as cancer) is a matter of "luck" more than their own role. Middle-class participants, however, showed a stronger sense of their personal involvement in determining their fate. They talked more about fighting the illness they had.

Issues of childbirth and social class have received less attention. A few social scientists (e.g. Nelson, 1983; Hurst & Summey, 1984; Martin, 1992; Davis-Floyd, 1992, 1994; Lazarus, 1994; Zadoroznyj, 1999; Kabakian-Khasholian et al., 2000), however, have shown that social class plays a significant role in how women perceive childbearing and the extent to which they wish to have control over their pregnancies and births. Emily Martin's work (1990, 1992) is situated well within the analyses of Blaxter (1990) and Blair (1993). Martin (1990, 1992) has shown that social class impinges on women's perceptions and expectations of their births and bodies. The issue of control was the most salient for middle-class women. These women sought control of themselves as they labored and gave birth and resisted medical control. Working-class women, however, rejected the idea of self-control, but focused more on their lived experience of childbirth such as the intensity or length of labor pain.

The work of Ellen Lazarus (1994) contains a similar suggestion. She showed that lay middle-class women were concerned with making choices that would allow them to have some control over their pregnancies and childbirth. To ensure this control, the women chose their own doctors to act as their advocates within the health-care system. For middle-class health professionals, they were also concerned with issue of control, but their knowledge of the system was exercised as a way of maintaining that control. For poor women, however, they "neither expected nor desired control but were more concerned with continuity of care" (1994: 25). Lazarus (1994: 26) admits "choice and control are more limited for poor women, who are overwhelmed with social and economic problems."

Maria Zadoroznyj's recent work (1999) explores the issues of power, identity, and control in childbirth among working- and middle-class Australian women. Her research suggests that women's attempts at control over the management of their first births are markedly influenced by their social class. Middle-class women were able to exercise choice and control more than the working-class women and this, Zadoroznyj (1999: 284) argues, is because the middle-class women's material resources "enable choice." To begin with, in their birthing career, middle-class women were more "active seekers" and working-class women tended to be more "fatalistic." For both groups of women, a number of changes took place in attitudes and sense of self, following the experience of first birth. But, for the working-class women, cultural resistance became much more evident than for the middle-class women. Clearly then, Zadoroznyj's research shows that cultural resources such as education, social milieu, and material resources play major roles in shaping the characteristics of obstetric encounters.

What makes the middle-class women behave so differently from their working-class counterparts? Following Pierre Bourdieu's theoretical framework of "habitus" (1977), I argue that individuals' choices and sense of control are determined by their social positions. Habitus, according to Bourdieu (1977: 95) is "an acquired system of generative schemes objectively adjusted to the particular conditions in which it is constituted, the habitus engenders all the thoughts, all the perceptions, and all the actions consistent with those conditions, and no others." To Bourdieu (1984), the habitus is embodied in the context of social positions of people. This indoctrinates people into a lifestyle that is based upon their position. And hence, it serves to reproduce people's existing social structure. Simon Williams (1995: 599) argues that, "it is in the relationship between habitus and capital, located within the context of the different social fields of society (i.e., the relationship between position and disposition) and the struggle for social distinction, that lifestyles are constructed." Individuals from different social classes may then have their own "logics of practice" (Bourdieu, 1990) and "tastes" (Bourdieu, 1984), by which I mean "choices" that fit their social positions. For some, their lifestyle choices, or "choice of necessary" (Bourdieu, 1984), may be limited, or even made impossible, by their economic and social constraints. Even if people have a similar goal to achieve, such as giving birth, their actual experiences and their levels of control are likely to be very different according to their social class memberships (Williams, 1995: 597). As Bourdieu (1984: 172) contends, "life-styles are thus the systematic products of habitus, which . . . become sign systems that are socially qualified (as distinguished, vulgar . . .)". To put it simply, to Bourdieu, as Williams (1995: 597–8) suggests, "it is the (class-related) habitus which, through taste and the bodily dispositions it engenders within particular social fields, together with the volume and composition of capital, determine not only lifestyles and the chances of success in the symbolic struggles for social distinction, but also class-related inequalities in health and illness." Adding to Bourdieu and Williams' argument, I contend that due to inequalities in access to and choices of health care, we witness an unequal struggle in empowerment and control between individuals (and here I mean the women from different social class backgrounds) in society.

SOCIAL CLASS, CHOICE,
CONTROL, AND RISKY SELF

Although existing literature has suggested that women's social positions influence the extent to which they passively accept or actively reject medical technologies (Kabakian-Khasholian et al., 2000), I contend that self-perception of
"risk" among women, regardless of their social backgrounds, plays a significant
role in their acceptance or rejection of medical interventions. The literature suggests that it is the middle-class women who have a tendency to reject medical
interferences including the use of medical technologies. It is a means whereby
women show that they are able to manage their own bodies and this, as a result,
empowers many pregnant women (Romalis, 1981; Oakley, 1986; Martin, 1992;
Lazarus, 1994). The work of Robbie Davis-Floyd (1992, 1994), however, reveals a rather different notion of empowerment and self-control. Davis-Floyd
(1992, 1994) points to differing attitudes and perceptions of childbirth interventions, which she calls the technocratic model of birth, among middle-class
background women in the United States. In her study, 70 percent of the women
were not only excited by, but also "comfortable with their highly technologised
obstetrical experience" (Davis-Floyd, 1994: 1128). These women did not express their interests in resistance. Rather, they seemed to actively seek, and
were empowered by, the medical interventions in their birth. Noticeably, these
women occupied high-status positions of prestige and authority. These women,
Davis-Floyd (1994: 1128) points out, "seemed to see technology as integral to
all areas of American life, and they fully expected that the very best in the modern technology of the body would be brought to bear on their pregnant bodies
and the fetuses within them in order to ensure that their births were competently
managed and controlled, and therefore, safe." To these women, choosing to
give birth with the assistance of technology provided them with a sense of control. One woman, for example, "preferred the sense of control provided by a
caesarean, and in no way saw this as a disempowering loss, but only as an empowering gain because it was something she had caused to happen" (Davis-
Floyd, 1994: 1131). Davis-Floyd (1994: 1136) concludes her findings that these
women are "far from resembling the passive victims of technocracy . . . all were
active agents in their birthgiving, albeit in radically different ways—and in their
relationships, pro or con, to the hegemonic technocratic model." Curiously
enough, for these women, Davis-Floyd (1994: 1136) points out, "that agency
took the form of control."

Theoretically, Davis-Floyd points to the notion of risky self among the
middle-class women in her study. Her findings sit well within the interpretation of self-identity within the conditions of high modernity (Giddens, 1991).

Anthony Giddens (1991: 80-81) argues that "high modernity is future-oriented, a society of experts rather than oracles, and a world of 'risk' in which we need constantly to remake ourselves." Hence, "high modernity forces choices on members of society." Gidden's work is applicable to my interpretation of childbirth in "modernised societies where a variety of discourses depict the process as an inherent risk and where different experts claim to have the truth" (Zadoroznyj, 1999: 273). The concept of risk has intruded into many areas in the postmodern world (Beck, 1992; Olin Lauritzen & Sachs, 2001), and the world of childbearing is no exception (Lane, 1995; Liamputong et al, 2003). Giddens (1991: 182) acknowledges that "by acknowledging risk the individual is forced to accept that any given situation could be one of those cases where 'things go wrong.'" Childbirth, clearly, could go wrong at any given time.

How then do individuals attempt to deal with risk? Simon Carter (1995: 142) suggests that as individuals live within the modern period, they may attempt to "manage the problem of danger by attempting to constitute boundaries that [are] then controllable . . . via the application of scientific rationality as useful and beneficial to decision-making." In this sense then, as Carter (1995: 142) puts it, "dangerous uncertainties are excluded by being made knowable." The discourse of risk in childbirth, as I shall demonstrate in this chapter, may make women attempt to manage it with a caesarean section. Women may come to believe that if they know exactly what will follow through having a caesarean, birth then may not be that dangerous.

Under the conditions of high modernity, structural inequalities previously articulated continue to exist. As Anthony Giddens (1991: 6) puts it, "class divisions and other fundamental lines of inequality, such as those connected with gender or ethnicity, can be partly defined in terms of differential access to forms of self-actualisation and empowerment." As I shall show in this chapter, the social class of the women influences their perceptions of self risk, and hence, determines the level of their choices and control in childbirth.

SOCIAL CLASS AND CHOICES OF BIRTHING CARE

Choices of hospital of birth and doctors among the women in this study were not homogeneous. Eight middle-class women received care from private obstetricians. These obstetricians operated in either a private hospital or a private section of a teaching hospital. Six rural women gave birth in a local public hospital with no private obstetricians. Eight rural and seven urban middle-class women had their babies in a public teaching hospital in the city.

Most rural poor women received care from public doctors at public hospitals. Only a few had their private obstetricians at public hospitals. Due to their financial constraints, most rural poor women did not have the same access to continuing care as did their middle-class sisters. A few rural women who could afford to pay chose to give birth in a maternity hospital in Chiang Mai City as they believed that a city hospital would have more medical technologies than their local one. In addition, the local hospital admits all kinds of patients, some of whom might have highly contagious diseases and could endanger the well-being of their babies. These women would travel into the maternity hospital in the city for the sake of their babies. Hence, there were also costs of travel involved in this. As Payao, a rural woman, remarked:

> I went to the maternity hospital in Chiang Mai City as people told me that there would not be too many diseases in that hospital as it is only for the mothers and babies. If I went to our local hospital or other public hospitals, there would be a lot of diseases around as there are many patients with different diseases and as we have to mix with them, the chance of getting some diseases would be high.

Sinjai, an urban middle-class woman with a good education, actively chose her own private obstetricians for both births. She also chose the best hospital in Chiang Mai at the time of her pregnancy. This, she believed, would ensure that the baby would be safe and she would be looked after better.

> When I had my first child, [X] hospital was the best hospital in town. And when I had my second child, [Y] hospital was the best, as it has every thing and it was very convenient and comfortable for me. Even the room was very good. My doctor worked there as well.

Women who had private care, even though the birth was in a public hospital, were able to have their own doctor present at the birth. Sirin, an urban woman, had her private doctor in a private hospital.

> I was able to choose my own doctor, as I had the baby in a private hospital. The doctor told me that he would be the one who delivered the baby. He told the nurse to fetch him when my labor started, and he did come to deliver the baby for me.

Similarly, Ruchira, a rural woman, was fortunate to be able to choose to give birth in a private hospital, as she believed that doctors in private hospital were friendlier than those public hospitals. In addition, women had strong beliefs in a doctor who would pay more attention to a patient in a private sector.

SOCIAL CLASS AND THE
LIVED EXPERIENCE OF VAGINAL BIRTH

Women's birthing narratives reveal differing experiences between those of rural poor and middle-class backgrounds. Many of the rural poor women were not very vocal about their birthing experiences. They tended to say that their births were not too traumatic, but not too easy either despite the fact that there were many opportunities for them to articulate their birth experiences during the interview processes. Most would simply say that their births were "normal" and not much to talk about. However, one woman, Srinang, who had a breech birth, compared a difficult birth with being tortured. She elaborated on her birth experience:

> The birth was not long, but it was torturing. As it was my first birth, it was so painful. I had great pain on the lower abdomen. And the pain, it was difficult to say what it was like. All I could say was it was like being tortured.

Due to the breech birth, the doctor recommended a caesarean, but later changed his mind as he believed that the baby was small enough to be born vaginally. It is worth noting that Srinang was a public patient in a local public hospital. Her class status might impinge on the doctor's decision. Caesarean births entail more costs on the part of the women, and public patients like Srinang may be seen as lacking financial support to pay for the service.

On the other hand, most of the urban middle-class women would express their views at length. Their narratives showed that some women experienced a difficult birth. Darunee, an urban educated woman, had a difficult and long labor as her baby was large. After the birth, she also hemorrhaged. She believed the hemorrhage was due to the size of her baby.

> My birth was a horrific experience, as the baby was big and it was difficult to deliver him. It took him a long time to descend and my cervix did not open properly. Then after the birth, I was hemorrhaging. The nurse told me that I lost so much blood that they had to put me in an ICU for a night. The birth of my baby was not easy at all.

Obstetric interventions seem to be prevalent among the women who experienced a vaginal birth. Noticeably, these interventions were more prevalent among urban middle-class women. Induction was the most common experience for these women. Warunee, an urban woman undergoing her first birth, told us:

> As soon as I got to the hospital and the nurse informed my doctor about my condition, he ordered an induction straight away so that my cervix would open. He said my labor was in an advanced stage and the baby needed to come out very soon.

Many women went through vacuum suction, as Sumalee, an urban uneducated woman undergoing her first birth, said:

> I had my baby naturally but he was sucked out. His head was too big and I didn't have enough strength to push him, so the doctor used suction.

It is also notable that women consented to obstetric interventions due mainly to their concerns about the well-being of their fetus. But, on a closer examination, recommendations by doctors seemed to have more weight on women's decisions. When asked how she felt about the forceps and vacuum, Sumalee, an urban educated woman who had her own private obstetrician, remarked:

> I was worried about the safety of my baby, I was afraid he might not be safe as they used a machine to suck his head out. I felt that the baby's head was far away from my pelvis, like he was floating inside me. So, I was worried about it.

When asked if the doctor explained to her about the need for the vacuum, she said:

> My doctor said that because I didn't have strength to push. He said I had to push harder as the baby didn't descend enough and because of this, he needed to use a machine to suck him out. Also the baby's heart beat was slow too. The doctor was worried about the baby, and that is why he used suction.

Similarly, Sirin, an urban woman, was advised to have suction. She was worried about the well-being of her baby, but eventually consented to the doctor's recommendation, as he said it would be dangerous for the baby without the suction. Wasana, an urban woman, also needed suction for the birth of her baby. She had difficulty pushing the baby, as the baby's head would not descend. Her doctor then suggested a vacuum suction to which she agreed, as she was concerned about the well-being of her baby. This lithotomy was also practiced in the private sections in a teaching hospital where most middle-class women gave birth. Sumalee told us about the birth position:

> I gave birth lying on my back. When I felt the pain, I lifted my bottom and the nurse told me not to do so. I think we all have to give birth only in this one position. I think it is for the convenience of the doctor. This is a private sector that I am talking about. What would it be like if you give birth in a public section! I think we could imagine it, don't you!

Nevertheless, regardless of the women's social backgrounds, episiotomy was common among women who had vaginal birth. Both rural poor and urban middle-class women were given similar treatment. Isara, a rural woman, told us that:

> When I was in labor, the doctor cut my vagina and this hurt a lot particularly when I went to a toilet. I could not sleep for 2 to 3 nights due to the pain. It was

like I wanted to pass my feces. I was so confused about the pain as I just felt pain all over my body.

Similarly, regardless of their social backgrounds, all women gave birth lying down on a labor bed with their legs strapped to the metal (lithotomy). Their arms were also strapped so that they would not move too much when the contractions were strong. To these women, their birth experiences were degrading and disempowering. Warunee, an urban woman, said:

> I gave birth with my legs separated apart, just as what women have to do in hospitals. The doctor would tell us to lie on our backs and our legs are separated on the metal stuff. Even our arms, they will be tied up so that it would prevent us moving around too much.

CHOICE, CONTROL, AND RISKY SELF: MAKING SENSE OF CAESAREAN BIRTH

Out of thirty women I interviewed, eleven underwent a caesarean section. Of these eleven women, three were from rural poor and eight were from urban middle-class and educated backgrounds. Only five of these middle-class women had their second birth via caesarean and two had repeated caesarean sections. This section is inevitably a reflection of the middle-class women's voices as they experienced more caesarean births than rural poor women. What made women consent to caesarean birth? Three main themes were apparent.

Self-Identity and Sense of Control

For some middle-class women, it was because of their previous pregnancy outcomes, in Anthony Giddens's words (1991: 143) "a fateful moment," that acted as a catalyst for choosing a caesarean birth. Maria Zadoroznyj (1999: 279) argues that, "women's self identities changed in ways reflected in their behavioral approach to subsequent births." As such, "identifiable turning points occur in individual life trajectories." This was particularly so for women who had lost a child. Wilai, an urban educated woman with a nursing background, elected caesarean for the survival of her fetus. Her first baby was born by induction. He was very weak after birth and died soon after. Due to this loss, Wilai decided that her next child would not have to go through a traumatic event as had her first child. In addition, the second baby was rather large in relation to her own small body. These factors made Wilai determined to have a caesarean birth despite advice from her obstetrician to first try vaginal birth. She elaborated:

> I thought a lot about choosing caesarean because I was worried about the well-being of my baby. If I had a big body, I might try to experience childbirth pain as most mothers have to go through. I wanted to know what it would be like to experience pain in childbirth. But, I was afraid that I might lose the baby through childbirth process, so I decided to have a caesarean instead of vaginal birth. My doctor said if he was me he would try a vaginal birth and if things did not go well then I could have caesarean. But, I did not wish to try to risk my baby's life, as I have lost one already.

As Robbie Davis-Floyd (1994) suggests, choosing a caesarean section is seen as having a sense of control. Wilai too perceived it this way. She believed that by choosing her own birthing method she was able to control the safety of her baby. This became clear when she was prompted with her feelings of not having a natural birth for her second birth. She elaborated:

> I thought about this a lot. I weighed my decision to have a caesarean with so many things. For one, I am a small person and I might not be able to push the baby. I was concerned about the baby. If I was big, I would have liked to touch on the feeling of pain of a natural childbirth as other mothers would have so that I would appreciate what it was like to be a mother giving birth. I wanted to have that experience too, but I was worried that I might lose my baby so I decided to have a caesarean instead.

She made her decision despite the fact that many of her colleagues (nurses and academic nurses) prompted her to attempt a vaginal birth. She said:

> Many people said I should not have a caesarean section; I should have tried a vaginal birth first and if it was too difficult then I could have an emergency caesarean. But, I thought that why should I go through childbirth pain and then have pain from an operation again. No, I don't want two lots of pain, so I decided to have caesarean birth from the beginning.

Women's sense of control was also clear when they discussed their choice of day and time for a caesarean section. This trend has also been found among Chinese in Hong Kong (Reichart et al., 1993; Lee et al., 2001; Yip et al., 2002). As in the Chinese culture, astrology plays an important role in shaping Thai beliefs and behaviors (see Naksook & Liamputtong Rice, 1999). Astrology is used to foretell an individual's long-term future and characteristics. Since people are born at different hours of the day, different days, months, and years, their future life and characteristics are different. Some days will be more favorable than the others. A person who is born on Tuesday, for example, is foretold as:

> A brave spirit, prone to quick anger and unyielding to others. Will be a strong support to parents and family but annoyed by some relatives. Intelligent, kindly

spoken and active; must move elsewhere to succeed. Trouble will come in two periods. But, will achieve a prosperous and peaceful old age (Wales, 1983: 5).

In my study, these characteristics were clearly important to many of the middle-class women and their families. Wilai, an urban educated woman, talked about the decision she and her husband made to select a date for a caesarean as follows:

My husband wanted the baby to be born on either a Monday or Thursday, but not on a Saturday. He said a Monday child will be clever and smart and if a baby is a boy he will become a soldier. A Thursday child will be a strong child and easy to raise. A Saturday child will have a dominant fate which means that he or she will be stubborn and may become aggressive and parents will have problem in bringing them up. The baby was due around Thursday and because my doctor's schedule was not too busy on Thursday, we chose a Thursday.

In Wilai's case, her choice and sense of control was complicated by the fact that she lost her first child after birth. In her mind, if she had had a vaginal birth, then she would let nature take its course; she would not interfere with nature. However, since a caesarean birth allowed her to have a choice, she then wished to choose a day which would be good for the baby so that the baby's chance of survival would be greater.

I had a bad experience with my first child. We did not pay attention to anything. Whenever the baby wanted to be born, let it be. But when he died, we looked for something for us to be able to rely on, so that was what we did, choosing a birth date for our baby. We would do anything to make the baby live.

A few rural poor women who elected caesarean births tended to believe that it would be easier to give birth by such a method. In addition, caesarean reduced prolonged pain, so it would not be too traumatic. For these women, it was a way for them to control and manage their own bodies. When asked how she felt about having a caesarean operation, Pimjai said:

Because the labor pain was so tremendous, and when the doctor said he would cut me, I just told him to go ahead with it. I said whatever you wanted to do, even you put me on a chopping board [operating table] just go ahead. The pain was too much for me to bear; it was like being tortured, and so I wanted the doctor to operate on me, so that I would be able to manage with my labor pain better.

Risky Self

The notion of risk was also prominent in the women's narratives about the need for a caesarean section. At one level, risk related to the consequence of not taking an action to prevent any future negative birth outcome. Women chose or agreed to have caesarean operations as a means to avoid any risk which might be posed to the well-being and safety of their babies. Nida, an urban educated woman, had her second birth via caesarean section despite her intention to have a vaginal birth like her first birth. When asked why this happened, she remarked:

> The labor took too long; it was longer than ten hours that I was in labor and the baby would not come out. My doctor examined the cervix and said it opened too slowly. Also the baby was very big. I did not want to take any risk, so I asked him to give me a caesarean section.

Prapaporn, an urban woman, also agreed to have a caesarean section, despite her resistance at the beginning, as she was concerned about the safety of her baby.

> When the pain was too great for me to bear, I said to the doctor whatever you wished to do just do it as long as my baby was born safely. I didn't feel afraid of the operation any more, even though I thought I would try vaginal birth as much as I could do so.

Srinang, a rural poor woman, had a breech birth. The doctor first recommended that she needed a caesarean section but later decided that she should attempt a vaginal birth. When asked how she felt when her doctor recommended an operation for her breech presentation, Srinang remarked:

> I would be afraid of the operation but at the same time I might have to agree with the operation because the baby was in a breech position which would make the birth difficult and might be dangerous for the baby. So, even though I would be afraid, I would have the operation. I thought the operation would be good for the baby's safety.

The probability of 'personal risk' was also seen as a possibility of having a caesarean birth. This was more so among rural poor women. Women talked about the history of caesarean births in their family that might contribute to their self risk of having caesarean births. Women believed that their chance of having a caesarean birth would be higher if their mother had had a caesarean. As such, caesarean birth might not be avoided; it was something beyond one's control. Lakana, one of the three rural poor women who had a caesarean section, was convinced that her risk of having a caesarean birth was high.

> The probability of caesarean births runs in my family. My mother had three children. I was the only child who escaped a caesarean delivery. My sisters were born by caesarean. When I was pregnant I anticipated caesarean birth, as the

chance was very high. My baby was not big at all. He weighed only 2900 grams; not even three kilos. For some babies, even though they weigh more than three kilos, they do not have to be born by caesarean section.

Perceptions of Risk and Trust in Medical Knowledge

The narratives of many middle-class women revealed that the most common and prominent reason for having a caesarean birth was a recommendation by their doctor. It was clear that women had trust in medical knowledge due to their self-perception of risk. Some women mentioned their age as a reason for a caesarean section. Siriporn, an educated urban woman who had planned for vaginal birth, was told by her doctor that she was rather advanced in age to have vaginal birth and this would be too "risky." He asked if she would consider a caesarean section. She consulted her husband who was concerned about the size of her pregnancy. He believed the baby was too large for her to attempt vaginal birth. This suspicion was also confirmed by the doctor who found that her pelvis was too narrow. All these prompted Siriporn to elect a caesarean section for both births. Despite her initial attempt for a vaginal birth, she believed her doctor's advice had more weight than her own knowledge.

Siriporn's narrative also revealed that the notion of "once caesarean, always caesarean" was prominent in the Thai health-care context. When asked for her reason for caesarean birth of her second child, she said "because my first birth was caesarean, the second one will have to be caesarean too. So, the doctor organized a caesarean section for both births." Manee, a rural educated woman, also had repeated caesareans. Her first caesarean was performed in a public hospital. Her second birth was in a different public hospital and a doctor made an arrangement for a caesarean section.

Some women mentioned their own bodily malfunction as a potential self risk and a reason for the doctor to recommend caesarean. Araya said her pelvis was too narrow and the baby did not turn, hence, her doctor advised a caesarean. Patanee, an educated urban woman, also was told that her pelvis was too narrow and that she needed to have a caesarean section. She elaborated:

> My doctor told me that my pelvic outlet was narrow and I would not be able to give birth vaginally. I intended to give birth vaginally, but when the doctor told me that I would have a difficult birth due to my narrow pelvis and I would have a long labor and experience a lot of pain, I thought I had to follow his advice. And also, I was thinking about the safety of my baby too. If I tried a vaginal birth, I might cause some problems. So, I agreed to have a caesarean; to put the matter into the doctor's hands might be safer for the baby.

Patanee intended to have a vaginal birth. But, when the doctor advised her to have a caesarean section, she agreed. When asked what prompted her to change her mind, she remarked:

> I had great fear about giving birth by myself from the beginning. But if there was not any complication with my birth, then I would try to give birth myself. I did not ask for a caesarean birth at the beginning. However, I had problems so I decided that I should put my fate in my doctor's hand as he would know what to do and it would be safer.

Lakana, a rural uneducated woman, was advised to have a caesarean birth due to her physiological deficiency too.

> The doctor said my pelvis was too narrow and the water did not break and the baby's head did not descend . . . The doctor checked my pelvis three to four times and he said if I left it like that [attempting vaginal birth] the baby would die. So, I had a caesarean.

CONCLUDING DISCUSSION

What can we make of the women's accounts of their childbirth experiences? In this section, I attempt to put their narratives into four main themes: women's lived experiences of childbirth and social class; social class and obstetrics interventions; alternative views of caesarean births; and risk and childbirth.

Childbirth, Social Class: Women's Lived Experiences

This chapter clearly shows that social resources such as financial resources and education play a salient role in shaping the embodied experience of birth among women in Northern Thailand. Women's narratives show that the "everyday lifestyle," or as Pierre Bourdieu (1984) calls it the "habitus," concerning middle-class women's control over the experience of childbirth of differs somewhat from that of the rural poor women. As Maria Zadoroznyj (1999: 284) suggests, middle-class women's material resources enable choice. This is particularly so for their deliberate selection of a medical technology. For the middle-class women, the idea that they can exercise choice and control is at the center of their orientations and practices. In Zadoroznyj's study (1999), the middle-class women chose medical interventions, such as pain relief, to allow the control of pain and hence of their own behavior as a way to express their sense of self-control.

The middle-class women in my study tend to be more vocal about their embodied experience of birth than their rural poor counterparts. Was it because of their class position that women feel empowered enough to be vocal? Or, to put it another way, would it be because the rural poor women are more fatalistic in their orientations and practices as suggested by Mildred Blaxter (1990) and Alan Blair (1993) and hence, they tend to accept whatever happens to them? Or, is it because of their marginal "habitus" that renders them voiceless in birthing care?

Following the theoretical concept of the "habitus" of Bourdieu (1984), Marsha Hurst and Pamela Summey (1984: 621) argue that a woman's choice of birth is determined by her social position. In addition, her choice of health practitioner means choice of the type of care she will receive, as we have seen throughout childbirth history (Wertz & Wertz, 1977). Working-class women, as Margaret Nelson (1983: 296) points out, have limited opportunities to make choices. What these women receive in childbirth tends to be outside their control. In my study, choices of doctors and places of birth are clearly dictated by the women's social positions. Middle-class women have more financial resources to enable them to actively seek care from private doctors or doctors whom they believe they can trust. Rural poor women have fewer choices in where they should give birth, the type of doctors they can see, and of the hospitals that cater to their needs. This may also contribute to their voicelessness, as they may not feel empowered enough to make their voices heard.

Social Class and Obstetrics Interventions

From the Thai women's birthing narratives, it appears that obstetric interventions abound in Thai birthing care. In the last few decades, Thailand has undergone modernization. One consequence of this is that birth is medicalized, as in other western societies (Martin, 1992; Davis-Floyd, 1992, 1994; Zadoroznyj, 1999; Riewpaipoon et al., 2005; see also chapter 2 in this volume). Obstetric interventions permeate hospitals, private or public. Some of these interventions, such as artificial rupture of membranes, episiotomy, lithotomy position, and forceps and suction are now seen as dangerous to the mothers to be (Nelson, 1983; Zadoroznyj, 1999). But, all these are still practiced in Thailand (see chapter 4 in this volume). It is not surprising then that we found that women of all social classes were treated with similar medical technologies/interventions. It seems, as William Arney (1982) suggests, that medical professionals, including obstetricians, have power and their power is eminently embodied in the prevalence of interventions used in hospital births.

Previous literature suggests that obstetrical intervention varies by social class. Margaret Nelson (1983) found that working-class women had births marked by more medical intervention and less personal participation than middle-class women. Accessing health care is also determined by women's social classes. Dona Glei and Noreen Goldman (2000) found in their study of pregnancy-related care in rural Guatemala that poor indigenous women were unable to access high-cost options such as private doctors for pregnancy care or private hospitals due to low socioeconomic status of the women. In linking rates of caesarean birth to class positions, Marsha Hurst and Pamela Summey (1984: 625) suggest that financial resources are the main reason for the higher rates of caesarean birth among middle-class women. I have demonstrated in this chapter that this is also true for many of the middle-class Thai women. More middle-class women were the target of the intervention than were their rural poor sisters. It seems that their financial resources render them to have more contact with medical interventions. On the contrary and with a few exceptions, the rural poor women are unable to pay for these interventions. As such, the woman's habitus influences the doctors' recommendations as to whether she should have medical interventions.

Embracing Caesarean Birth: Alternative Views

Existing feminist discourses suggest that middle-class women wish to have control of their own bodies and births. Hence, these women tend to reject medical interventions as a way of showing that they are able to manage their body, and this empowers birthing women (Martin, 1992; Lazarus, 1994). In my study, as in Robbie Davis-Floyd's (1994), this seems to be a contradiction, that middle-class women see caesarean births and medical interventions as something providing them with a sense of control that empowers them. To these women, control, as Lourdes Campero and colleagues (1998: 401-402) suggest, "is more a matter of having participated in and having followed the evolution of their labour."

Robbie Davis-Floyd (1994) has shown in her study that many of the middle-class women deliberately chose the technocratic model of birth as a means to exercise control over the uncertain process of childbirth. The middle-class women experienced medical technology "as a liberation from the tyranny of biology, as empowering them to stay in control of an out-of-control biological experience" (Davis-Floyd, 1994: 1137). These women manipulated medical technology to control their own bodily experience. To these women, because they participate "in a society's hegemonic core value system . . . [they] are most likely to feel empowered by and to succeed within that system" (Davis-Floyd, 1994: 1137). As such, as Maria Zadoroznyj (1999: 270) suggests, women chose to use "technocratic childbirth in empowering ways." The middle-class women in my study perceive and behave similarly, and they perceive caesarean birth in a positive light.

Occasionally, however, for some poor women, they are not just "passive victims" of their material resources. No matter how little resources women have, they make use of them. Women can be "active actors" who have their own aims and reasons for using or not using these medical technologies (Denny, 1994, 1996; Malin et al., 2001). This is what I found. Some rural poor women had caesarean births as a means of controlling their own bodies and births. Despite some financial constraints, some women would travel to the city to have the better birthing care they wanted. They too seek health care by which they can have control over their body and birth.

There are some other possible explanations why women in my study embrace caesarean birth. The woman herself may come to believe that the professional's medical knowledge is the best for her (Jordan, 1997). It seems, as it has recently been pointed out in the notion of "public trust" in health care (Straten et al., 2002; Riewpaiboon et al., 2005), that women may be confident that they will be adequately taken care of when they are in need of health care. Women may also have trust in the "fiduciary ethic" (Gray, 1997) of their doctors; that their doctors will put the women's interests above their self-interest. In addition, the medicalized discourse in Thailand's health care, like childbirth in many Western societies, sees childbirth as "potentially pathological" and that "something can go wrong at anytime" (Lazarus, 1994: 27–28). This has put women under the control of medical professions. As Ellen Lazarus (1994: 27) succinctly puts, if women do not do "everything" like following doctors' advice, it is their responsibility if they do not have a "perfect" birth, or a healthy baby, and they will be blamed for it. This is a powerful message that pregnant women receive. It is not too surprising then that women come to believe that their doctors know best about their pregnancies and births, and that they have to rely on medical knowledge to ensure that they have done everything possible to ensure a healthy birth, such as agreeing to undergo a caesarean section (Lazarus, 1994). Maria Zadoroznyj (1999: 284) demonstrates in her study that the presentation of self among working-class women was "as a self with little knowledge, little choice and considerable faith in medical 'experts.'" I, however, found that this faith, or trust in Bradford Gray's term (1997), in medical experts permeates both the rural poor and the middle-class women's narratives. Although many of the middle-class women have adequate knowledge and choice, they still have faith in their doctor's medical expertise and knowledge.

As childbirth is "a technocratic service that obstetrics supplies" (Davis-Floyd, 1994: 1127), medical practitioners may be keen to perform a caesarean section due to financial incentives (Hurst & Summey, 1984). Jeffrey Gould and others (1989) found in their study that caesarean sections were higher in suburban hospitals where most women were insured. In Thailand, doctors' incentives to perform caesarean may be the consequence of receiving the higher fee charged, including a higher gratitude fee (Hanvoravongchai et al., 2000). It is worth noting that nearly all in this sample who had caesarean births were urban middle-class women. This confirms high rates of caesarean sections among middle-class women in Thailand (Hanvoravongchai et al., 2000) and in other regions (Barros et al., 1996; Belizan et al., 1999; Murray, 2000; Potter et al., 2001). Emily Martin (1992) too points to the dominant pattern in America that women in higher socioeconomic classes receive substantially more caesarean sections.

Risk and Childbirth

Risk discourse in the women's narratives of caesarean embodiment is also apparent. Caesarean birth, for some women, may be seen as "having rescued the fetus from some menace, usually brought about by their own maternal deficiency" (McClain, 1990: 208). To these women, caesarean birth may be perceived as "a straightforward cultural good" because it "offers pain free birth and the baby is safe, as doctors can assist in it" (McClain, 1990: 208). To these women, Carol McClain (1990: 208) argues, caesarean birth does not signify "the loss of control over one's own body." Rather, caesarean operation "corrects for biological deficiencies and failures that cannot be controlled by other means." This empowers women to have faith in themselves and have a sense of control. Gerardo Zanetta and colleagues (1999: 147) found in their study, that for women in Italy, vaginal birth was "symbolically related to the fear of possible risks to the fetus." Some believed that intervention procedures would reduce risks for the mother and her baby. In addition, caesarean birth was seen as "a painless mode of delivery, compared with the 'terrible' pain related to vaginal delivery."

Additionally, the women live in the risk culture of modernity (Giddens, 1991; Beck, 1992). In this condition, Anthony Giddens (1991: 123-124) theorizes, "for lay actors . . . thinking in terms of risk and risk assessment is a more or less ever-present exercise . . . The risk climate is thus unsettling for everyone; no one escapes." As Ulrich Beck (1992) points out, we now live in a "risk society." Robbie Davis-Floyd (1994) takes a step further arguing that because we now live in a society whereby biomedical/technocratic discourse of birth is dominant, we are bound by risk discourse. The technocratic model, according to Davis-Floyd (1994: 1125) is a "cohesive hegemonic mythology . . . [which] . . . functions as a powerful agent of social control, shaping and channeling individual values, beliefs and behaviours." The essence of this discourse is "separation of humans from nature, of mind from body, of mother from child. Such conceptual distinctions are implemented through ritual acts that produce physical embodiments of the underlying worldview" (Davis-Floyd, 1994: 1126). As such, in the case of childbirth, the physical embodiment of birth is produced through ritual acts of caesarean sections. Under this technocratic discourse, Davis-Floyd (1994: 1127) argues: "the female body is viewed as an abnormal, unpredictable and inherently defective machine. During pregnancy and birth, the unusual demands placed on the female body-machine render it constantly at risk of serious malfunction or total breakdown." Maria Zadoroznyj (1999: 268) too points to the power of this discourse that "can be explained by its success in constructing birth as a situation of inherent risk requiring expert technical management by specialist obstetricians." Birth, defined as a risky endeavour, "legitimates and increases the probability of the excessive intrusion of technological interventions in an arguably 'natural event'" (Zadoroznyj, 1999: 269). It is not too surprising then that the women in my study embrace this risk in their birthing experiences; not only risks that may be imposed on their births, but also risks to their babies.

But notions of risk differ between the women. As Simon Carter (1995: 134) points out, risk may mean very different things to different individuals in different contexts. Mary Douglas (1990: 2) suggests that, although risk is a "technological reification of the word 'danger,' risk was a relatively neutral term, taking account of the probability of losses and gains." Thai women in my study clearly thought of risks in term of probability; something that may or may not happen. But, their risks, or probability of risks, are related to the history of a caesarean in the family. It seems to be a common belief among Thai people that if a mother has a caesarean, the chances are that her daughters will have caesarean births too. This is not heredity, but probability. Zygmunt Bauman (1993: 200) points out that the word risk "belongs to the discourse of *gambling*, that is to a kind of discourse which does not sustain clear-cut opposition between success and failure, safety and danger." Carter (1995: 135) too suggests that "risk alerts us to uncertainties about whether the future is safe or dangerous." Hence, "the idea of risk points simultaneously to the presence of and possibility of danger" (Carter, 1995: 136). To the women in this study, their perceptions of risk addressed their uncertainties that the births might be safe or dangerous. To reduce these uncertainties, a caesarean as a possibility of security was chosen. This line of thinking was also noticed by study with Thai women living in Australia (see Liamputtong & Naksook, 1998a).

In sum, then, my research indicates that the lived experience of birth differs between individual women and women of different social class backgrounds.

As feminist writers (Oakley, 1979; Croghan, 1990; Martin, 1992; Smart, 1992; Lazarus, 1994; McMahon, 1995; Luke, 1996; Zadoroznyj, 1999) have advocated, differences between women need to be taken into account in providing care to women in childbirth so that sensitive and appropriate birthing care for women can be achieved.

Chapter Four

Giving Birth in a Hospital

ﭏ

Almost everywhere in the tribal world women birth either sitting, kneeling, or squatting, with a helper supporting and massaging them from behind or in front, or with other means of support taking the place of the helper.

(Goldsmith, 1990: 32)

INTRODUCTION

Childbirth in many developing countries has become increasingly medicalized and professional delivery in a medical environment is increasingly being promoted (Kabakian-Khasholian et al., 2000). Under the medicalization of childbirth (as opposed to the quote given above), care provided to women, as Lourdes Campero and colleagues (1998: 396) put it, is undertaken "exclusively by doctors and nurses who generally consider labor and childbirth as potentially pathological conditions for which the mother and/or child require specialized and technological care." Within this framework, health-care providers stand out as key agencies in childbirth. Some writers maintain that the focus on medicalized birth, all too often, leads to problems associated with medical dominance, poor communication between health-care providers and the women, and impersonal treatment in hospital births (Kabakian-Khasholian et al., 2000; Phillips, 1996; Liamputtong & Naksook, 1998b; Yelland et al., 1998; Rice, 1999a; Small et al., 1999, 2002). Due to this, feminist writers have demanded the right of women to choices about childbirth and criticize "overmedicalization" of childbirth in the West (Arney, 1982; Martin, 1992; Cunningham, 1993; Davis-Floyd, 1992, 1994; Lane, 1995; Zadoroznyj, 1999).

73

In the last two decades, women's voices concerning birthing care in Western societies have been documented (see for example, Martin, 1992; Davis-Floyd, 1992, 1994; Brown et al., 1994; Lane, 1995; Zadoroznyj, 1999). However, the voices of women who reside in developing countries have only recently received attention. Tamar Kabakian-Khasholian and colleagues (2000), for example, examined Lebanese women's experiences of maternity care. Women in their study, the authors claim, had total trust in their doctors. Women seldom questioned the usefulness of many routinely applied procedures. Many aspects of the technical care were intimidating and the women experienced discomfort with these procedures. Women also valued good interaction with their doctor. The researchers also found that the extent of passivity and feelings of discontent women had varied according to their social class and the amount of psychosocial support they received throughout the process of childbirth.

As a result of modernization or Westernization of Thai society, childbirth in Thailand has also become medicalized (Muecke, 1976; Whittker, 2000, 2002; see also chapters 2 and 3 in this volume). As in other societies, childbirth in Thailand has increasingly moved from a familial and social domain to that of hospital-based medicine, for many an unfamiliar institutional setting and knowledge base (Liamputtong Rice & Manderson, 1996). The medicalization of childbirth, in turn, has resulted in a highly technological approach with routine hospital procedures (Muecke, 1976). But, how Thai women at the present time, and particularly women living in the Northern Thai context, perceive and experience childbirth is largely not known.

In this chapter, I firstly discuss women's embodied experiences of their childbirth in hospitals including issues related to choices of hospitals, birth position, obstetric interventions, and family members at birth. Secondly, I look at issues relating to length of hospital stay and postpartum care of the mother and her newborn infant. Women's satisfaction with care in the hospital is then discussed. Lastly, I offer some theoretical understanding of the women's embodied experience of childbirth in Thailand.

CHILDBIRTH EXPERIENCES AND CLASS: PASSIVITY, CHOICES, OR SATISFACTION

As I have discussed in chapters 2 and 3, the social class of women determines choices of childbirth as well as their desire to follow medical advice during pregnancy (see also Nelson, 1983; Martin, 1992; David-Floyd, 1994; Lazarus, 1994; Zadoroznyj, 1999). Women who have better education and employment are, for example, in a better position to seek private care from their own medical practitioner. Unlike their urban middle-class counterparts, to working-class and poor women, access to special care is denied and they have to rely on public health care. To poor women, issues of choice are not an option. Poor women are, therefore, as Ellen Lazarus (1994: 26) states, "constrained by the conditions under which they have babies and the kind of care open to them."

According to Lazarus (1994: 29), as I have pointed out in chapters 2 and 3, "taking control of one's life and body is a middle-class perspective." She argues that the women's class, education, and financial positions enable them to have an active say in their childbirth experiences. This is, however, denied to those rural poor women, who are restricted by limited knowledge and overwhelmed with economic problems. Hence, they have limited choices and control over their pregnancy. Emily Martin (1992) also maintains that poor women tend to be cooperative with the medical profession in a hospital setting. Women are less likely to express their concerns and anxieties than middle-class women. Poor women, then, tend to be characterized by their passivity (Kahakian-Khasholian et al., 2000).

Lyn Quine and colleagues (1993: 111) examined satisfaction with birth experience of middle- and working-class women in England. They too argue that working-class women tend to lack social support and adequate information: "they are less supported than middle-class women, and they lack adequate information about childbirth." Due to this, working-class women are less likely to see childbirth as a rewarding experience. Ann Oakley and Lynda Rajan (1991) too point out that working-class women often lack social and emotional support. This may be one reason why they may tend to feel dissatisfied with their birth experience.

Tamar Kabakian-Khasholian and colleagues (2000) suggest that similar class distinctions also characterize women in non-Western societies. Their work highlights issues of self-control among women in Lebanon. Lebanese women's perceptions of the obstetric care they received were generally characterized by the feeling of passivity. But, the extent of their passivity and the desired level of personal control over the process of childbirth differed according to the women's social class. For middle-class women in Beirut, the feeling of subordination to the medical profession is less apparent than that of women from the other areas. Women in remote rural areas have less demanding attributes despite the accessibility of prenatal care. This may be due to their low social class and low educational level as compared to women from Beirut. As Lazarus (1994) suggests, the middle-class women in this study are more likely to demand personal choice and lessened professional dominance over their childbirth process (Kabakian-Khasholian et al., 2000: 111).

In this chapter, the discourses of women's childbirth experience in hospitals will sit alongside these theoretical frameworks.

EMBODIED EXPERIENCES OF BIRTH IN HOSPITAL

Women's embodied experiences of childbirth in hospitals reveal four discourses: choices of hospital of birth, birth position, obstetric interventions, and family members at birth.

Choices of Hospital of Birth

All women except one gave birth in a hospital. One rural poor woman delivered her baby at home, but the newborn's umbilical cord was cut in a hospital. When asked for the reason why she gave birth at home, she articulated that:

> I started to have abdominal pain at night but the baby was born at 7 in the morning. We were all in chaos trying to organize me to get to the hospital, but the baby just popped out. So, my aunt had to fetch a car to take me to the hospital to have the cord cut. We tried to ask the doctor at the local hospital to come to cut the cord, but he refused to come out. He said as a patient, we had to go into the hospital. (Saengchan)

Regardless of women's social background, they all believed that hospital birth was safer than homebirth which was a common practice in the old days in Thailand, especially in the North. Often, women articulated that there were sufficient modern medical technologies and doctors were skillful and had medical knowledge to assist them in childbirth if any complication arose. It seems that women had more faith in the modern hospital setting than in their own home environment.

I have pointed out in chapter 3 that there were differences in choices of hospital of birth and doctors among the women in this study. Six rural women gave birth in a local public hospital with no private obstetricians. Eight rural and seven urban middle-class women had their babies in a public teaching hospital in the city. Eight middle-class women received care from private obstetricians. These obstetricians operated in either a private hospital or a private section of a teaching hospital.

Most rural poor women received care from public doctors at public hospitals. Very few had their private obstetrician at public hospitals. Due to their financial constraints, most rural poor women were denied the same access to continuing care that their middle-class sisters had. Some rural women who could afford to pay chose to give birth in a maternity hospital in Chiang Mai

City, as they believed that a city hospital would have more medical technology than their local one. Orachorn remarked that she chose to travel to the teaching hospital in the city because:

> I went to that hospital because they had appropriate equipment and the maternity building was separate from other patients. My local hospital did not separate patients; women who are giving birth have to mix with other contagious patients.

Family Member at Birth

It is a common practice in Thai public hospitals that a woman's husband or other family members are not permitted to be present at birth. All of the women in my study who attended public hospitals, even a teaching hospital, stated that they did not have their husband with them at birth. Many wished to have their husband present, as Ruchira, a rural woman, commented:

> When I had a baby, there was no one from my family with me. The hospital would not allow anyone in. But, I wanted my husband to be there for me as he would be able to give me emotional support when I was in pain.

Sira, an urban woman, made a request to her private doctor that her husband should be present at birth, as she believed her husband needed to see how difficult is was for a woman to give birth as well as to provide her emotional support at a critical time. But, the doctor did not agree. She reiterated:

> My husband was not at birth. I asked my doctor during antenatal check up if my husband could be in the room with me, but he was jokingly said "Don't let him in there because when he sees your blood, he will faint."

In some private hospitals as well as private sections of public hospitals, however, the presence of a husband was possible. In my study, there were only a few women who attended a private hospital but a few more gave birth with a private obstetrician in a teaching hospital.

> When I had my baby, my husband was in the labour room with me. I was in a private section of [X] hospital. My husband was allowed to be in the room with me, to give me emotional support. He held my hand when I was in labour. I felt secure to have him in there as he was my emotional support. He only held my hand, as he didn't know what else he could do. He kept his eyes on me and I noticed his eyes were watery. He probably was scared too as he could see how traumatic I was giving birth to a baby. (Sumalee, an urban woman).

But, some women felt considerate of their doctors, as the presence of their husbands might obstruct the work of their doctors. The women, hence, would ask their men to stay outside even though their husband might wish to be present at birth. Wilai, an urban educated woman, had her baby in a public hospital and wished to have her husband present as:

> I wanted him to give me emotional support. Also, he is a father of my baby so I wanted him to be the first person to see the baby. But, I thought his presence might mess up the hospital routine, so I asked him to stay outside. If I had the baby in a private section, I think he could go in with me.

Wilai's husband too wished to stay with her in the birthing room, but Wilai was afraid that his presence might interfere the hospital system; meaning that the hospital staff might find it difficult to work around him. She decided to ask him to wait outside the birthing room.

Some urban middle-class women were fortunate enough to have their colleagues who were academic in the teaching hospital or a nurse practicing in the hospital where the woman gave birth present for emotional support. This was denied to rural poor women who lack such a privileged network. Wilai, an urban educated woman, had a friend who was a nurse, at the birth with her. She said:

> I had my friend in the room with me. She is a nurse there. Outsiders are not allowed in the birthing room. As my husband is an outsider, I didn't feel that I could ask him being there with me.

Siriporn, an urban educated woman, had her colleague who was an academic teaching in the hospital present during an epidural caesarean. The presence of her colleague was a great support to her, as she was fearful of a caesarean operation. But, the presence of her colleague meant that she would not be able to have her husband with her.

> My friend asked if I wanted my husband in the theatre with me but I said it was not necessary for him to be there. He could just wait outside. I was considerate about having too many people in the theatre. My friend was a nurse at that hospital and all of her nurse friends came in to see me. So, there were too many people in there and if my husband was in there too, it would have been too many for the doctor to cope.

Prapaporn, an urban woman, had two of her colleagues stay with her during birth. When asked to articulate how she felt to have someone she knew present at birth, she remarked that she felt confident and more certain about the birth as she had an epidural caesarean.

Many rural poor women, however, wished to have their mothers present at birth more than their husbands. Saengchan, for example, put it this way:

I wanted my mother to be in the birthing room with me, as I missed my mother in time of difficulty and my mother would take good care of me too. When I was in the birthing room, there was no one with me as the hospital would not allow anyone in there.

It was interesting to note that when rural poor women were asked if they ever wanted to ask to have their husbands present at birth, nearly all of them remarked that they would not "dare to ask" or "too afraid to ask." It seems that their social position in the society as rural poor and uneducated women in comparison to those of health care providers contributed to their lack of self assertion, even if it was for their own emotional well-being.

There was one exception, however. Orachorn, a rural poor woman, commented that the reason that family members were not allowed to be present was that their family would not be able to do anything. The presence of a doctor would be sufficient for any birth.

No one from my family came into the birth room with me, as the doctor would not allow them. But, even if they could come in, what could they do anyhow. They could not do anything. I think having a doctor close by would be much better. All the family members can just wait outside.

LENGTH OF HOSPITAL STAY

Length of hospital stay varied depending on the method of birth women had. For those who had a caesarean section, most stayed for five days or more. For women having a vaginal birth, most stayed between two to four days. There were two women who stayed only one day and four who stayed over six days. One stayed one week due to problem with hemorrhage and one for two weeks due to her diabetic condition.

A common practice in a Thai hospital is that if a woman has a vaginal birth, she should stay only three days. For a caesarean birth, it may be four days or longer, but usually around five days. Araya, an urban woman, had a caesarean and stayed for five days. She was told that it was time to go home when she left the hospital. Prapaporn, an urban woman who had a private obstetrician in a public teaching hospital, was asked if she wanted to go home on the sixth day. The doctor told her that if she was ready to go, then she could go home. As she felt that both she and the newborn were healthy and strong enough, she told her doctor that she would go home. Naree, an urban poor woman, stayed in the hospital for two days only and she went home because the doctor told her that she was strong enough to go home. However, Saengchan, a rural poor woman, only stayed in a local hospital for one day. She asked to go home early, as she did not have any health problem or a tear.

Some women, despite having a caesarean birth, might go home early if the doctor believed that both the mother and baby were well. Wilai, had a caesarean birth with her second child, and stayed in hospital for four days only. The reason to go home, as she remarked, was:

> The baby was with me and he seemed to be strong. My abdomen was alright. I could eat alright. And the pain was not too great; I could endure it. So, we could go home.

Most women would go home according to the recommendation of their doctor.

> I stayed in hospital for four days. I was ok. I had no fever or anything and the baby was healthy and strong enough. So, the doctor told me that I could go home, that it would be better for me to take care of the baby at home and the weather would be better there too. (Warunee)

Sumalee, an urban woman, stayed for three days and her reason for going home was that:

> I stayed three nights and two days in hospital; the night I gave birth and two days afterward. The hospital has a policy that if you have a vaginal birth, you can only stay 2 nights and 2 days, then you should go home. The doctor came around to check me and the baby and said that we both were healthy and strong enough to go home.

When asked if she ever asked to go home herself or to stay in hospital longer, she said that she only did what was recommended by the doctor.

Nonetheless, there were few rural women who would ask the doctor if it was time for them to go home. For these women, the need to observe a traditional confinement practice known as *yu duan* (see chapter 5 in this volume) was seen as essential for the recovery and well-being of a new mother. Essentially, a new mother must confine herself to home and keep the body warm by wearing long trousers, long-sleeved top, socks, and a scarf on her head and neck. During this *yu duan* ritual, she has to consume certain foodstuffs prescribed for a new mother and she must not expose her body to any coldness such as a cold shower and wind. The women in the study commented that if they could go home early, they would be able to commence the postpartum ritual sooner. For other women, they believed that home environment was better for them and their newborn. Being more convenient for family members to take care of them at home was also mentioned as a reason for going home early. As Darunee, a rural woman who gave birth in a public hospital in the city, put it:

I stayed in hospital only two days. I felt a bit bored there and as I could help myself and I felt that it would be better for me to go home and take care of my new baby at home as it would be convenient for me to do things I needed to do like *yu duan*, so I asked the doctor if I could go home earlier.

POSTPARTUM CARE OF THE MOTHER AND NEWBORN

There are two salient findings regarding postpartum care of the new mothers and their newborn infants.

Treatment of the Perineum—The Use of a Spotlight

As all women who had vaginal birth delivered in a horizontal position, it is not too surprising to see that all of them had a tear or a cut (episiotomy) requiring stitches. Women mentioned that a doctor and nurses would instruct them about how to take care of their episiotomy wounds. The most commonly mentioned instruction was to keep the perineum clean by washing it with warm water. If there was any pain, the women would be given some pain relievers.

In Northern Thailand hospitals, at least in Chiang Mai where this study was undertaken, using a spotlight to help heal an episiotomy wound is a common practice. A nurse will place a spotlight close to the vagina and cover it with a blanket for at least ten minutes, twice a day; but for some women there may be several times each day. It is believed that the perineum will dry out quickly and properly. Women mentioned that when this was being done, the perineum felt comfortable. Warunee reiterated that:

> A nurse used a spotlight to shine on my vagina so that the tear would get dry very quickly. She would wash the tear and then use the spotlight. I was in the hospital for four days and the nurse would do that for me every day, once per day.

Sinjai, an urban educated woman, also had a spot light when she had her first baby by vaginal birth. She said: "the nurse shone the spotlight on my vagina to make the cut dry. I felt that when she was doing it, the pain was reduced." Similarly, Naree, an urban poor woman, told us:

> The doctor cut my vagina when I had my last baby and some stitches were done too. They would clean the cut and dry with a spotlight. They put the spotlight near my vagina and cover it with a blanket. The cut would be warm and dry quickly. I felt comfortable when it was done on my vagina.

Isara, a rural woman, also had the spotlight during her stay in hospital. She remarked when asked how she took care of the cut:

> The doctor dried the wound for me. It was done about 10 minutes twice per day; one at 6 am and another one at 6 pm. The doctor used a spotlight to dry it.

Isara continued to do so at home too, as it was easy for her to do so. She had her mother who assisted her with the activity. She elaborated:

> After I went home, I also did it as we could manage so. I used a reading lamp in stead of a spotlight. I lied on my bed and my mother held the light on my vagina for me. She also placed a blanket on my bottom part to trap as much heat as possible, so the cut would get dry quicker. I continued this for 10 days until the cut was dry properly and I had no more pain on the cut.

Rooming-In and the Care of a Newborn

The teaching hospital in Chiang Mai practices a rooming-in policy (Yimyam, 1997). Essentially, all women were expected to take care of their newborn babies during their hospital stay. After birth and after being briefly put on the breast, the baby would be taken away in order to allow the mother to rest. The mother would be asked if she was ready to have the baby. Once the baby was brought back to the mother, she was expected to take care of her own baby. Sumalee elaborated that:

> After the baby was born, the nurse brought it to me so that I could put her on my breasts for a while. She then took the baby away but later on came back to ask if I wanted my baby back. I said yes as I wanted to see her. So, she brought the baby to me and since then until we left the hospital I was expected to take care of my baby.

During this period, a new mother would also be taught about breastfeeding and taking care of her newborn.

Noticeably, for the women themselves, most did not wish to take active care of their newborn babies. When asked to articulate their perceptions of rooming-in, most mothers said they preferred the nursing staff to take care of their babies. Warunee, an urban educated woman, put it this way:

> I did not ask the nurse to bring the baby for me. I thought the nurse should take care of the baby as then I was still in pain from childbirth and I could not really even take care of my own body. I wanted to have some rest after giving birth, you know. For me, the nurse took the baby to me in the morning and I had to look after him since then.

Sumalee, an urban woman, was asked if she wished to see her baby not long after birth. She said she would. However, once the baby was brought to her, the nurse did not take the baby back again. For Sumalee, then, she had to look after her baby throughout her hospital stay.

SATISFACTION WITH CARE

Women expressed their satisfaction with birthing care in terms of birth outcomes. As long as they could bring forth a healthy baby, they felt satisfied. Additionally, women's satisfaction with care was determined by the level of interaction with their caregivers. Sumalee, an educated urban woman, for example, had a long labour and the doctor suggested vacuum suction. The doctor explained to her that suction was essential in her case, as she did not have strength to push the baby out and the baby's heart rate was low. Sumalee felt that she was informed in the birth process, and hence, agreed to the suction despite her fear about the well-being of her baby. Sirin, an urban woman, also had satisfactory experience with her doctor. She too had to undergo vacuum suction. She described her experience:

> It took too long for the baby to be pushed out so the doctor recommended suction. At first, I was afraid about the procedure as I thought it might damage my baby. But, the doctor gave me good explanations and he said he would do his best not to cause any danger to my baby. He said too that if the suction was not used, then the baby might be in danger. So, I agreed to the procedure.

It appears that women had their trust in their doctors when seeking care. Ruchira, a rural woman, agreed to have vacuum suction despite her fear about the harm that it might cause on her baby. When asked how she felt when the doctor told her that the baby needed suction, she put it this way:

> I was afraid that the baby might be in danger, but I felt confident in the doctor. He possessed knowledge of getting the baby out by suction, so I trust that he would be able to help me.

Some women, however, were unhappy with the care and services they received in hospital. Payao, a rural woman, had her baby in a public hospital in the city and experienced poor treatment by her caregivers. She was left on the labor bed alone for too long. This is what she told us:

> They just left me there to give birth by myself. I would tell other mothers that if they want to have a baby, don't go to this hospital. They put me on the bed, told

me to lift my legs and then they strapped me on the metal straps. They told me
to push the baby out. None of the doctor or the nurse paid attention to me at all.
They were two nurses there but they just left me like that.

For Payao, the presence of health-care providers such as nurses and a doctor
would be a source of emotional support at a critical time like birth. This un-
satisfactory experience, however, had prompted her not to return to that hospital again.

For some, bad attitudes of health-care providers during the labour process
were expressed as the cause of their dissatisfaction with care. Prapaporn, an
urban educated woman, was scolded by a midwife while she was strapped in
bed during her labour, as she was not relaxed enough for the midwife to feel
the baby's head. She elaborated this experience that:

> I was put on the labor bed with my legs strapped as the nurse was preparing for
> the birth of my baby. She scolded me when she could not feel the baby's head.
> She told me to push and relax. I thought I did. I was taught to relax during birth
> so that the birth would not be quick and I thought I was not tensed at all. I was
> puzzled when the nurse said so. The doctor could not feel the baby's head but it
> was my fault. As the pain started to be more intense, I did not pay much atten-
> tion to what she said to me.

One rural woman had difficulty giving birth and the baby was born via forceps. The baby's arm was dislocated, but she was not informed about this. It
took her several months to notice that the baby could not use her arm properly. Only when she took her baby for a checkup did she learn about the
tragedy. She, however, felt that she could not do anything about the doctor's
performance, as she did not find it out when she was still in the hospital. She
also felt powerless to challenge her doctor due to her lack of education and
status. Her sense of powerlessness was only expressed when she had the opportunity to talk about it when she participated in this research.

CONCLUDING DISCUSSION

The women's narratives reveal that childbirth was managed within the medical system. Contrary to what Majorie Muecke (1976) found several decades
ago that just over half (51.7%) of Northern Thai women gave birth in hospitals, all women (except one) in my study had their babies in hospitals. In fact,
what I have found is that the women in this study wished to have professional
delivery in the hospital setting. It is clear that the women in this study, similar to women in other parts of the world (Kempe et al., 1994; Kahakian-

Khasholian et al., 2000), gave safety as the primary reason for their choices of birth in hospitals. In a study with pregnant women in England, women chose hospital-based births because of their fear about the risk of unforeseen complications that may occur during the birthing process (Johnson et al., 1992). Recently, Tamar Kahakian-Khasholian and colleagues (2000) also showed that women in Lebanon seek hospital births because they believed it was safer than homebirths.

What can explain this popular belief? Clearly, as I have suggested in chapters 2 and 3, due to the modernization or westernization of Thai society, childbirth in Thailand has become medicalized (Muecke, 1976; Riewpaiboon et al., 2005). The medicalization of childbirth, in turn, has resulted in a highly technological approach with routine hospital procedures (Muecke, 1976; Rothman, 1989; Martin, 1992; Jordan, 1993; Lazarus, 1994; Ram, 1994: Davis-Floyd, 1994; Lane, 1995; Campero et al., 1998; Zadoroznyj, 1999; Riewpaiboon et al., 2005). Childbirth within this medicalized framework is seen as a medical problem and it can only be handled by medical professionals such as doctors and nurses in hospital settings. Defining birth as such it becomes "an event controlled by more or less anonymous specialists carrying out standardized techniques on a woman's body" (Muecke, 1976: 379). In most industrialized countries, childbirth is seen as a disease state, a physical bodily disturbance (Cosminsky, 1982: 225); the woman's body is the subject of control by medical professionals and technology (Martin, 1992; Davis-Floyd, 1993, 1994; Lane, 1995; Zadoroznyj, 1999). A woman is required not only to give birth in a hospital where she may have little or no control, but she is also given the message, as Davis-Floyd (1997: 497) points out, about her powerlessness, "defectiveness," and her dependence on science and technology (Liamputtong Rice & Manderson, 1996: 5).

As Majorie Muecke (1976: 381) found several decades ago, Thai women in Chiang Mai adopted the Western model of birth because they "perceive it as much safer, as reducing the risk of death during delivery." Women also believed that doctors can help in time of difficulty with birth due to their "esoteric knowledge," Western medications, and modern equipment used in hospitals (Muecke, 1976: 381). To the women, hospital birth then provides them and their newborn babies with extra protection.

Women's embodied experiences with hospital birth reveals the "passivity" discourse (Szasz & Hollenger, 1956). As Tamar Kabakian-Khasholian and colleagues (2000) have shown in their study, women accord total trust to their doctors and very rarely question the many routine procedures in hospitals. What can explain this passivity? Straten and colleagues (2002: 227) point to the essentialism of "public trust" in health care. Accordingly, public trust in health care is "defined as being confident that you will be adequately treated when you are in need of health care; this means confidence in the agency re-lation between patients and health care providers" (see also Mooney & Ryan, 1993; Bluff & Holloway, 1994; Gray, 1997; Gilbert, 1998; Mechanic, 1998; Mechanic & Meyer, 2000; Riewpaiboon et al., 2005). As patients, Lucy Gilson (2003: 1457) contends, public trust in health care "provides the basis for our judgment that health care providers will act in our best interests." As such, as Straten et al. (2002: 228) suggest, public trust in health care can be perceived as "a way of enabling people to deal with the uncertainties and risks associated with handing their fate over to health care providers" (see also Misztal, 1996; Gilbert, 1998). As childbirth is seen as critical life event and individual women do not know beforehand the outcomes of their preg-nancies, women may hand over control of their situation to health care providers. As Gilson (2003: 1459) suggests, "trust in providers may matter more to vulnerable patients with higher risks," such as women in childbirth. As childbirth is a life crisis event, women giving birth may have a higher level of trust in their caregivers than other users of the health care system. Muecke (1976: 381) too points out that Thai women in the North would leave the close support of their families to give birth in a lonely place in a hospital and tolerate the invasion of their bodily privacy because they believe that "doctors know best."

However, the passivity of the women in the study may be due to, as Campero and others (1998: 396) suggest, the medicalization of childbirth. Un-der the medicalized birth, the medical staff has authority due to their esoteric knowledge (Muecke, 1976: 381; Bluff & Holloway, 1994; Jordan, 1993; Davis-Floyd & Sargent, 1997; Zadoroznyj, 1999). As Rosalind Bluff and Immy Holloway (1994: 163) succinctly put, it may be that women have been encouraged to hand over responsibility for childbirth to health professionals. And hence, "this unquestioning acceptance may lead to a model of passivity in which the women accept passively what is done on their behalf." Additionally, within the medicalized birth, "the encounter takes place in an environment which is unfamiliar to the patient; the patient must adopt physical positions which are uncomfortable, passive, and dependent; and the communication is either scant or very complicated due to the jargon used." Women do not feel that they have the right to express their concerns or doubts. Rather, women en-ter hospital "feeling that they must be obedient and cooperative."

It seems that in Northern Thai hospitals, the involvement of women's part-ners is kept to a minimum. Not only did the women in my study passively ac-cept the hospital rules, some of them even become considerate of their doc-tors. It may be that women felt that they cannot behave as an "assertive consumerist" (Malin et al., 2001: 130; Wiles & Higgins, 1996; Lupton, 1997). This non-assertive behavior may be a reflection of the cultural stereotype of a passive role for both patients and for women (Parson, 1951). But, women may also feel that assertiveness may jeopardize their care received in hospitals as generally health-care professionals, particularly doctors, feel uncomfortable with complaining consumers (Allsop & Mulcahy, 1998) and demanding patients (Stein, 1990; Lupton, 1997: Malin et al., 2001).

It has been shown that social support during childbirth has its impact on women's experiences of birth, obstetric and birth outcomes, and the health and well-being of the newborn baby (Oakley et al., 1990; Quine et al., 1993; Campero et al., 1998). Lyn Quine and colleagues (1993: 107) suggest that, as childbirth is seen as a crisis or stressful life event, social resources function to "mediate the effects of stressful events on well-being" during childbirth. Social support is perceived as "the degree to which the basic social needs of an individual are met by means of interaction with others (Campero et al., 1998: 397). Emotional support in particular "refers to the behavior that brings a sense of comfort and makes a person feel that she is loved and that others are ready to take care of her and make her feel secure" (Campero, 1998: 397; see also Thoits, 1982, 1986). As Eleanor Holroyd and others (1997: 71) suggest in their study with Chinese women in Hong Kong emotional support from family members is important for women at the stressful time of childbirth. Marja-Terttu Tarkka and Marita Paunonen (1996) have also shown that a birthing woman's perception of the support provided by her caregivers such as midwives to meet her emotional needs during labor can enhance her coping efforts and positive feelings about her experience of birth. John Cunningham (1993: 482) too suggests that the sharing of emotional support with the husband and other support persons who were present during birth was valued by the women in his study with Australian women. He also maintains that the more time the women receive the support, the more satisfaction the women would have with their birthing care.

But, the fact that hospitals where most of the women in this study gave birth did not allow their partners or significant others to enter the labor ward, this as Lourdes Campero and others (1998: 396) contend, deprives women of the support they traditionally received from their families (see also Holroyd et al., 1997). In the old days, as Majorie Muecke (1976: 378) points out, "husband and wife are physically and emotionally united in intense effort to deliver their child." Thai husbands in the North have close involvement with childbirth, as this can be seen in a traditional way when men help women giving birth. But, now this has diminished, as husbands are not allowed to be present in a labor room. Under a medicalized birth, women's emotional needs and subjective experiences are ignored. Indeed, without the emotional support of their family members, the childbirth experience of many women becomes "a mechanical and intimidating process" (Campero et al., 1998: 396).

To counterbalance this, Eleanor Holroyd and colleagues (1997) suggest that family members, not only husbands, should be encouraged to accompany laboring women, but this would require changes to hospital policies. Marian Carter (2002: 437) too comments on the "positive health benefits" that husbands could provide for women through the added social support during birth. Carter (2002) suggests that men's involvement in childbirth may promote a better partnership between men and women. Arguably, Carter (2002: 438) puts, "pregnancy and birth are unique and carry special meaning as well as risks for the families involved," in particular for the woman's husband. I contend that this argument can be made with the women's situations in this study.

Although the length of their hospital stay was determined primarily by the medical outcome of their pregnancy (e.g., caesarean birth), women had different views about their hospital stay. Thai mothers' concerns were in many ways similar to those reported elsewhere (Brown et a, 1995; Liamputtong Rice et al., 1999). In Stephanie Brown and others' study (1995), reasons for going home early among Australian women included wanting to be with their families, being unable to sleep or obtain good rest in hospital, and not liking being in the hospital. In the study that my colleagues and I carried out with Thai immigrant mothers in Australia (Liamputtong Rice et al., 1999), however, we found that women would go home according to the hospital policy and being told by hospital staff, their dissatisfaction with hospital environment and food, and being lonely in hospital. Furthermore, family encouragement was cited as a reason to go home, as this would allow the women to commence their confinement practice sooner. The findings of my study confirm many points found in the Liamputtong Rice et al. study (1999).

Of interest among postpartum care provided in Thai hospital in the north is the use of a spotlight to help heal the episiotomy wound. Majorie Muecke (1976) argues that this is an adaptation of traditional practices of *yu duan* in the era of modernity (see chapter 5 in this volume). Muecke (1976: 381) suggests that one of the primary goals of the postpartum ritual *yu duan* practices is to dry out the uterus. It has to be noted here that in other parts of Thailand, a traditional practice of *yu fai* (staying-by-the-fire) ritual is observed by a new mother during the first thirty days after birth (Jirojwong, 1996; Liamputtong Rice et al., 1999; Whittaker, 2000, 2002). While observing this ritual, she must keep her body warm, by wrapping herself in a blanket, wearing a long-sleeved top and sarong or pants, wrapping a piece of cloth around her head, ears, and neck. This ritual has been referred to as a "mother roasting" ritual, a common practice in a number of Southeast Asian cultures (See also Manderson, 1981; Townsend & Liamputtong Rice, 1996; Liamputtong Rice, 2000a, b; Liamputtong Rice et al., 1999; Whittaker, 2000, 2002) and is regarded as vital to the well-being of a new mother. It helps to restore "heat" lost in childbirth, to flush out retained blood and placenta from the uterus, to make the uterus shrink to its normal size and to dry out the tear of the perineum. However, *yu fai* ritual is not observed in the northern part of Thailand. A new mother only observes *yu duan* ritual. *Yu duan* ritual requires all other aspects as in *yu fai*, except for the stay-by-the-fire aspect.

The adoption of spotlights in hospital may be due the fact that, as Muecke (1976: 381) contends, there is "some syncretism" between Thai tradition and Western models of childbirth in Thai hospitals. Health professionals in Thai hospitals appreciate the benefits of some Thai traditional practices, but somehow adapt the practice to suit the hospital equipment. As a spotlight is accessible in hospitals and elsewhere, the use of it to replace an elaborate ritual of *yu duan* is easily accepted. Although the women might continue to practice *yu duan* rituals upon returning home, the hospital attempt to incorporate a Thai traditional practice is warmly welcomed by the women in my study. I contend that the practice of spotlight in hospitals may not only practically assist them in the healing process, but also provides the women with symbolic ritual.

Women in general were satisfied with postpartum care received during their hospital stay. Maili Malin and colleagues (2001: 124) suggest that the women, as "an embodied subject, constructs the experience of birth in their interaction with others (here health professionals) within their socio-cultural context." Women may experience satisfaction or dissatisfaction in regard to different aspects of care. Their satisfaction or dissatisfaction is also determined by an important outcome measure such as a safe birth, or the processes of care. Vaida Bankauskaite and Osmo Saarelma (2003: 27), for example, show in their study with patients in Lithuania that consumers' satisfaction and dissatisfaction with medical services are determined by good relationships between doctor and consumers as well as information given during the interaction. Malin and others (2001: 124) too suggest that "one important part of patient satisfaction derives from a dynamic interactional process with medical personnel, the process of the treatment: how the care is given, what it includes, where it is given and by whom." This feeling of satisfaction, as Campero and colleagues (1998: 401) refer to, is the feeling of "being in control"; that is, women feel that they have the chance to participate in and follow their own birth process and this provides them a sense of empowerment. The women in my study made similar comments to these research findings.

However, there were some aspects of postpartum care that women were unhappy with. Of interest is that a number of women in this study commented on the rooming-in policy practiced in many maternity hospitals. Rooming-in practice as a routine policy in maternity hospitals was introduced during the 1940s with reluctance and resistance from some public health authorities, hospital administrators, and medical personnel (Jackson, 1948, 1953; Mandl,

1988). Once permitted, however, rooming-in has become a compulsory hospital routine (Rice, 1999b). As childbirth in Thailand has been medicalized, an adoption of rooming-in has also taken place in maternity hospitals (Yimyam, 1997). It is argued that rooming-in policy may help to create and strengthen the maternal-infant bond and establish breastfeeding quickly (Rice, 1999b). However, in my study (Rice, 1999b) with Southeast Asian immigrant women in Australia, it showed that many mothers did not perceive these as having the same importance. On the contrary, they believed that the policy placed a strain on them. Rooming-in created conflict between new mothers and hospital staff, due to cultural and role expectation differences. Women needed to observe their cultural practices including good rest and avoidance of physical activities, in order to regain health and strength after giving birth, but these practices are in contradiction with rooming-in policy. Since they had to participate actively in looking after their newborn, women felt that they could not rest properly, particularly at night, and several of them opted to go home early. These cultural and role expectation differences led to dissatisfaction with hospital care in many women. This is in line with what Peter Moss and others (1987) found in England. Mothers in their study felt the demands from the hospital staff on their involvement with their infants were too great and hence they felt dissatisfied with postpartum care. The women in Moss's study "preferred less involvement—doing less for the baby, getting more help and having less contact, particularly at night" (162). In Italy, Cuttini and colleagues (1995: 42) demonstrated that Italian mothers "appreciated the positive features of rooming-in, but also recognized its drawbacks." These drawbacks included difficulty in resting and tiredness, problems with handling the baby and interpreting the baby's cries. Cuttini and others (1995) concluded that despite the twenty-four-hour availability of rooming-in, women "always retain the possibility of having the baby in the nursery if they so choose." Stephanie Brown and others (1994) and Pranee Liamputtong Rice and colleagues (1999) have also documented similar findings. For the women in my study, although they wished to see their babies soon after the delivery, they would prefer the nursing staff to take care of their babies in the first day or so. The findings of this study suggest that there is a need to re-visit the rooming-in policy in maternity hospitals.

My data also suggest some differences between rural poor and urban middle-class women in terms of hospitals of birth, the opportunity to have a family member at birth and so on. It is clear that middle-class educated women are able to exercise their choices and control over their childbirth experiences much more than rural poor women. This confirms existing literature that women's social backgrounds influence childbirth experiences (Nelson, 1983; Martin, 1992; Lazarus, 1994; Zadoroznyj, 1999). It is, therefore, imperative that differences between women based on their social backgrounds need to be taken into account when dealing with Thai women in order to achieve sensitive birthing care for women.

It has been argued that women's satisfaction with their childbirth is determined by their involvement in making decisions concerning their childbirth and their sense of control over the whole process (Salmon & Drew, 1992; Beattie, 1995). As Arthur Kleinman (1980) and Robin DiMatteo (1994) suggest, communication between consumers and health-care providers plays an essential role in determining patient satisfaction. Women's voices are, therefore, essential if health-care providers wish to understand their wishes and needs (Kabakian-Khasholian et al., 2000). Judith Bruce's quality of care framework (1989, 1990) may be adopted for this. Among some of the fundamental issues of this framework, health-care providers need to be sensitive to women's concerns and provide women with ample opportunity to express them as well as respect for the women's rights to make decisions.

Childbirth, as Lourdes Campero and others (1998: 402) contend, is a stressful life event resulting from the "complex interaction between pain, immobilization, medical interventions, and the failure of interpersonal relations within health care institutions." I argue that care provided to women during birth needs to take into account women's emotional and subjective experience so that sensitive birthing care can be achieved. This will only make the childbirth of many women a more positive one.

Chapter Five

Yu Duan Practices as Embodying Tradition, Modernity, and Social Change

ϰ

The postpartum period is the liminal stage in a woman's passage through
the rite of childbirth. As in all such transitional stages, the person on the
threshold is in an extremely vulnerable position and must be segregated
from her community.

(Laderman, 1987: 174)

INTRODUCTION

The postpartum period has been identified as the most important period of
childbirth in cross-cultural studies (Pillsbury, 1978; Laderman, 1987;
Lewando-Hundt et al, 2000; Liamputtong Rice, 2000a, b; Whittaker, 2002).
In these cultures, a new mother is perceived to be in a stage of vulnerability
of harmful agents, natural and supernatural (Whittaker, 2002). Within these
cultures, numerous proscriptions and prescriptions imposing on a new mother
and her newborn during the postpartum period abound.

   Existing literature has pointed to the significance of traditional postpartum
practices in Thai culture (Hanks, 1963; Muecke, 1976; Mougne, 1978; Whittaker, 2000, 2002). We do not know, however, if traditional postpartum practices are still observed in Northern Thailand at the present time. As Thailand
has undergone modernization in the last few decades, I attempt to explore the
present pattern of postpartum practices in the Northern Thai context. First, I
explore the traditional postpartum beliefs and practices which still exist in
Northern Thai society today. Second, I examine the extent to which women
from different social classes adhere to traditions and their social support
which may hinder their desire to adhere to these. Third, I attempt to examine

93

the influence of modernization and medical dominance on traditions and the extent to which women have succumbed to this influence.

POSTPARTUM PRACTICES AS RITES OF PASSAGE: BECOMING A MATURE WOMAN

Existing empirical findings point to conceptualizing postpartum practices as rites of passage (Van Gennep, 1966). The postpartum period in many societies is seen as a dangerous, powerful, or polluting stage (Kitzinger, 1982). Following Victor Turner's theory (1967, 1979), Robbie Davis-Floyd (1992: 18) states that this liminality is the "stage of being betwixt and between, neither here nor there—no longer part of the old and not yet part of the new." The liminal periods are often connected with birth and death, the theory offers illuminating patterns of childbirth in many traditional societies (Turner, 1979; Davis-Floyd, 1992).

In rites of passage, people are separated from ordinary society. This can be seen clearly with women during the postpartum period. In most societies, parturient women are usually separated from normal social activities. A woman who has just given birth is vulnerable to dangers and illnesses due to her physical and emotional weakness caused by the act of giving birth. She is also capable of causing danger to others due to her perceived polluted nature of childbirth and its blood. The seclusion of rites of passage is, therefore, an attempt to safeguard the woman from danger as well as to protect others around her from her "liminal and polluted state" of health. Within this seclusion period, a new mother is taken care of by her close female kin in a separate room, or part of the house, where she does not have contacts with outsiders. Her diet and behaviors are monitored and modified throughout the seclusion period. The postpartum practice is seen as beneficial to women's health and well-being.

But more importantly, as Whittaker (2002) points out, postpartum practice bears "social significance." As Jane Hanks (1963) theorizes, the confinement period is not only perceived as care to protect a liminal woman from danger, but clearly serves as a rite of passage to mark the attainment of matured female status (Davies, 1994). By observing a confinement practice such as staying-by-the-fire in Thai culture, Hanks (1963:73) suggests, it "perfected her as a human being; restored and strengthened her body; improved her capacities as a nourisher, and strengthened her own *khwan* (soul)." Hence, her body is made mature by the fire's heating ritual observed during the postpartum period (Hanks, 1963). Whittaker (2000:147) contends that the confinement practice exits not only because of its health benefits for women, but also "because of the symbolic significance of the period of seclusion and regulation as a marker of female maturity." As such, postpartum practice ritually prepares women for their new status as matured mothers (Davies, 1994).

YU DUAN PRACTICE AS EMBODYING MODERNITY AND SOCIAL CHANGE

While a representation of a postpartum practice as a rite of passage provides an important cross-cultural understanding of the practice on women's health and status, I suggest that women's support network, their exposure to modernization and social change occurring in the society also have an influence on postpartum practices. Traditions are influential and authoritative. As I shall show in this chapter, many women hold on to their traditions. But, some actors may resist or attempt to alter them. Andrea Whittaker (2000) points to the degree of resistance among women in Northeast Thailand. Susan Bordo (1993: 193) too argues "even the most subordinated subjects are . . . continually confronted with opportunities for resistance, for making meanings that oppose or evade the dominant ideology." As Whittaker (2000) shows in her study of Northeastern Thai women, women make pragmatic choices about their childbirth practices and experiences and the discourse of modernity is adopted by the women to determine their choices. Very often, as Whittaker (2000: 11) suggests, the women explain their choices "in terms of differences between the past and the present, between modern life and past tradition." Closely relevant to this modernity discourse is the dominance of modern medicine on women's pragmatic choices.

In childbirth, including the postpartum period, Whittaker (2000: 42–43) suggests that Thai women are "experiencing a disjuncture between the 'traditional' values and expectations and 'modern' practices." Although the values women attributed to modernity and tradition are not uncontested, women seem to deal with the disjuncture "as personal dilemma" in their choices. And even though there are "tensions between 'modernity' and 'tradition,'" both continue into the present (Whittaker, 2000: 48–49). Women may identify themselves as being modern and hence relinquish their tradition and this creates their new identities as *samai mai* (modern) (Mills, 1999). But, this new self seems to be a prevalent discourse of urban educated women. Rural poor individuals remain marginal in the modernity discourse. As I shall show in this chapter, this can be seen clearly in the postpartum practices in Northern Thailand.

EMBODYING TRADITION

The Significance of *Yu Duan* Practices

The period after birth is considered to be the most vulnerable period of a new mother and of her life. For a period of thirty days, she is vulnerable to ill health and diseases. Hence, women believed that after giving birth they must be extremely cautious about their activities and diet. One grave consequence of this is that a woman will experience *lom pid duan*, which literally means wind illness caused by doing something wrong in the postpartum month. Minor symptoms of *lom pid duan* included thinness, weakness, and being easily affected by allergies. *Lom pid duan* may also manifest in bodily aches and pains. The aches and pains may appear in later life, but they may also appear soon after the confinement period is ended. A more severe symptom is manifested as *mao hua* or *jeb hoa*, dizziness and pain in the head. *Mao hua* normally makes the sufferers vomit. Additionally, *naen ok*, having a stuffy or choked feeling and pain in the chest, may be experienced. These two symptoms are caused by wind rising or pushing into the head and chest resulting in dizziness and pain. Most importantly, *lom pid duan*, according to the women in this study, is embodied as madness. Naree, an urban poor woman, said: "The symptom of women who are affected by *lom pid duan* is like a mad person. Her nerves are destroyed and this makes her insane." And if the woman is affected severely by *lom pid duan*, she may eventually die (cf. Symonds, 1991; Whittaker, 2000).

Lom pid duan can be caused by bad odors from foods or other things including perfume and soap. During *yu duan*, women must also adhere to certain foodstuffs. Any foodstuff which produces a strong odor such as lemongrass, spring onion, and *Cha-om* (*Acacia pennata*, a green vegetable that is typically used in Northern Thailand dishes) is to be avoided. Being exposed to cold water during *yu duan* is also believed to cause *lom pid duan*. This is referred to as *pid nam* or *pid neb cha*. As such, a cold shower is prohibited during the *yu duan* period. Malai also explained that most often if a woman breaks this taboo, the symptoms would appear when she is older (cf. Whittaker, 2000, for the practices in Northeast Thailand).

The Practices of *Yu Duan* Ritual

As in other cultures (Sich, 1981; Laderman, 1987; Chu, 1996; Symonds, 1996; Cheung, 1997; Liamputtong Rice, 2000a, b), during *yu duan* period lasting for one entire month (*duan*), a new mother must be confined to her bedroom or home. She must wear a hat or cover her head with a piece of cloth or scarf. She must wear a long-sleeved top, long trousers, and socks. All the windows and doors will be closed. This is to prevent the cold wind entering the body. Failure to do so may result in aching bones and bodily pains and other ill health in later life. As Saijai elaborated:

> During *yu duan* period, I must wear a hat and cover my head. I must wear a long-sleeved top and socks. Why do I have to do this? Well, my mother told me that the wind will get into my body easily if I don't do it. And this will cause pain in the bones. When I get older, I will get sick easily; I will be sick often.

Suriya cited the example of her sister who suffered from *lom pid duan* due to not dressing properly during *yu duan* period.

> I know this very well as my sister suffers from it. When she was in *yu duan*, she did not put on her bra and she went downstairs [still within the house]. She was wearing a short-sleeved top and had a long-sleeved top over, but she did not button up the long-sleeved top properly and the wind got into her chest. Even up to now [a few years past] whenever she feels the cold, she will be shivering and she can't have a cold shower at all.

A head is considered more vulnerable to coldness and wind. Therefore, it must be covered at all times. Malai, a rural poor woman, explained that a new mother must cover her head with a hat or scarf at all times, as failure to do so may cause pain in her head and this may further cause madness due to a prolonged head pain.

During *yu duan* period, binding of the abdomen is also practiced to help the uterus recover and shrink to its normal size. This will make the abdomen flat and tight and is referred to as *mod luuk kao ou* (Liamputtong Rice et al., 1999). Practically, the woman might use a piece of cloth to tightly tie her abdomen. This is commenced around two or three days post-birth.

> Binding of the stomach is very good. I have had 5 children but look at my tummy, it is still flat. The binding will help *mod luuk kao ou* and this makes the tummy flat quickly. I continued to do it even after *yu duan* finished because it made me feel good when I walked. If I did not bind it, when I walked I would feel that the uterus would drop and cause stomach pain. (Naree, an urban poor woman)

But, some women did not wish to do this, as it was too restrictive on their bodies. For others, particularly poor women, the practice became difficult. The material they used would not properly stay on their bodies, and as they had to keep working, it became difficult to manage. Malai, a rural poor woman, told us that:

> I did not do the binding so my tummy is still big now. Well, I did do it, but I did not do it all the time. It was too annoying as the cloth kept coming off. I tied it

and it would stay for a while and then it would get loose and fall off. Those who have plenty of money they can buy "Stay" or other belts to wear, so they could do so easier. I only used *pa kao ma* [cloth used by men in their daily routine], so it was easy to fall off.

Visitors are allowed during *yu duan*, but they should not be physically too close to a new mother. This was mainly due to their fear of smelling a bad odor. Malai, a rural woman, explained:

Visitors can come to see us during *yu duan* but they must be careful with the smell stuff. They can cause *lom pid duan* in a new mother. Like if they wear a perfume or their bodies are smelly, this will cause *lom pid duan*.

But, some women mentioned that this caution was mainly due to the fear of their own bodily odor. As they did not have a proper shower for a long period, their bodies would have some unpleasant odors, and these might offend their visitors.

Visitors, however, must be particularly cautious when visiting a new mother and her newborn. Suriya, a rural poor woman, explained the custom that:

Those who come to visit us, as they know that I am still observing *yu duan*, before they come, they would have had a shower to make their body clean. As they are afraid of causing *lom pid duan* in the new mother, they must make sure that their bodies will not have bad or strong smells.

As the woman's body is highly vulnerable during this period, visitors might not wish to visit them if they are ill. Women remarked that most visitors would know the customs very well. Only close relatives might visit the pair during *yu duan* period. Distant relatives and friends would normally wait until the *yu duan* period ended.

Gender of the Newborn and Length of *Yu Duan*

Gender dichotomy is pervasive in the women's accounts of life courses in Northern Thailand (cf. Mills, 1999; Fongkaew, 2002; Lytleton, 2002; Whittaker, 2002). It is a general consensus among the women in the North that length of *yu duan* is dependent on the gender of a newborn baby: male—*yu yon* (stay short); female—*yu yao* (stay long). The actual length varies, but in general, for a male baby, *yu duan* period is shorter than a female baby. Some women said for a boy, the *yu duan* period might last between twenty-seven to twenty-nine days and for a girl it should be thirty-one or thirty-two days. A few women mentioned twenty-eight days for boys and thirty-two days for girl; others said twenty-five days and thirty-five days. Some women mentioned even shorter days for boys and longer days for girls. Pimpan, a rural poor woman, stayed for one month and one week for her second birth, as she gave birth to a girl. She explained:

> They say for a boy we have to do it for 25 days to 28 days. This means we will exit *yu duan* before the end of the month. But for a girl, we are told to stay longer than one month. Perhaps, a girl is weaker than a boy and hence it needs more time to be with the mother. I think this is what older generations think about.

Women remarked that as a girl will bear more responsibilities and work harder during her lifetime than a boy, she deserves a good start in her life by having more contact with her mother during infancy. In Northern Thailand, weaving is traditionally seen as women's work, and weaving requires strenuous physical actions. It seems logical for the women that girls should be privileged during the *yu duan* period.

Pimjai, a rural woman, elaborated on the different length of *yu duan* that it has been a tradition in Northern Thailand. Older people had a saying for this longer length of *yu duan* for girls that "*pu ying—peua hook, peua fai*" (women—extra for weaving machine, extra for cotton) or "*pueu kan, peua gnan* (extra for work commitment). This is an intention for the girls that in the future they will have knowledge for surviving. For boys, there is a saying that "*pu chai—dtad kom hok, kom dab*"; meaning for a boy there is a need to break the sharpness of a spear or sword. So, the confinement is shorter. Symbolically, it must be short so that they will be easily taught and trained; that is to be easily controlled, and listen to parents, but not be too stubborn. It seems this belief is based on the fact that boys, when mature, will be out of control easily or will be likely to take risks more than girls (Fongkaew, 2002; Lytleton, 2002). However, this practice may be a reflection of the matrilineal practice which is still prevalent in Northern Thai culture, where women have a higher status than men (Potter, 1977; see chapters 1 and 6 in this volume).

Regardless of the length of *yu duan*, however, the logic of practice of *yu duan*, as women put it, was to ensure a close contact between a mother and her newborn infant. The prohibition of getting out and working was that the mother would devote the whole thirty days to her newborn. As she is not allowed, or expected, to perform any other tasks apart from taking care of her newborn and rest, the practice was logical because it allows the woman to be able to do so.

Despite this traditional rule, some women could not stay as required due to constraints in their lives. Wasana, an urban woman, only stayed twenty-five days for her first daughter as she was running her business and there was no one who could really running it for her. But, for her second child, which was a boy, she also stayed twenty-five days according to the rule.

Exiting *Yu Duan* Ritual

Exiting *yu duan* involves a series of ritualized procedures. The childbirth process is believed to make the body in a state of being "cold" and the body is opened up to harmful agents. At the end of the *yu duan* period, a new mother must undergo several rituals to counterbalance these. Traditionally, a steam bath method, referred to as the *hom ya* ritual is performed.

One method involves the use of hot bricks and medicinal leaves called *bai plao* (*Grawia paniculata*). Several leaves (around 30) of *bai plao* are piled up on several hot bricks. The woman sits on the leaves and hot bricks, and a blanket or sarong covers her body. She must say a prayer to make her wound heal quickly before sitting on the leaves. Once she sits on them, water is poured on the leaves to create steam. The heat and water in combination with the leaves create medicinal perfume for the woman to breathe in. The whole process is done in a bathroom or a closed room, and it usually takes about an hour. Some women mentioned using *pu leoi* (*Zingiber cassumunar*) instead of *bai plao*. *Pu leoi* rhizome is pounded and mixed with water. Several stones or bricks are heated and placed in a hole on the ground. *Pu leoi* liquid is then poured onto the hot stones and the woman sits on top of the hole. This will make the perineum dry and assist with the healing process. After this the woman will be showered with a herbal shower. The whole process usually takes about one hour or until the water is getting cold. Women mentioned that after taking this steam herb and herbal bath, they felt refreshed and as if the body has "opened."

Another type of *hom ya* ritual is also used at the end of *yu duan*. Essentially, a family member will boil a pot of medicinal herbs for the woman. Most mentioned herbs were mainly those from the citrus family such as tamarind, lemon, pomelo (shaddock; *citrus grandis*—much like the grapefruit), and *som bpoi* (a climbing plant of the genus Acacia, used medicinally) as well as *bai plao* and *pu leoi* rhizomes. The pot will be covered with a banana leaf and a hole in the leaf is made to let the steam through. It is then placed in front of her and she will bend her head down and breathe in the steam herbs. This will make her sweat. The sweat is to eradicate all poisonous essences in the body. The heat from the process is to assist the recovery of the uterus and close the body's pores so that the skin will be "tight." It is believed that if a woman has an aching head, *hom ya* will relieve the aching. These herbs can be purchased in a ready-made bunch from herbal shops. The *hom ya*, however, is prepared by the *mor muang*, a traditional herbalist, due to his knowledge of herbal medicines in confinement. These rituals appeared to be prevalent among women in rural areas, but a few urban educated women also practiced them.

The end of the *yu duan* period signifies the maturity of womanhood. Only after passing through this final stage does the woman emerge as a matured woman and hence her status has now been changed by motherhood (Hank, 1963; Whittaker, 2000, 2002).

SOCIAL SUPPORT DURING *YU DUAN*

Social support received during the postpartum period is significant in helping women cope with the upheaval of childbirth (Oakley, 1993; Moon Park & Dimigen, 1994; Rendina & Liamputtong, 2006). As commonly found in a more traditional society, most women in my study received support from their family members during the *yu duan* period. Most often women mentioned their mother and sisters as their prime support. Some had their mothers-in-law or grandmothers to help. Support from female members is crucial for the women in this study.

Remarkably, however, women made comments on the support of their husbands. Thai husbands in the North play many roles in childbirth, and the *yu duan* period is no exception. The men in the North are more involved with birth and the period after. The "universal proposition" theory of Sherry Ortner (1974) which suggests "woman is to nature as man is to culture" (Symonds, 1991: 268) is contested in this study. Ortner (1974: 75) argues that "giving life is seen as part of 'nature' and therefore devalued." But, as Patricia Symonds (1991: 269) suggests in her study with Hmong birth, "the creation of life is seen as a highly valued act both natural and cultural, neither one opposed to the other, for it is done by women and men. Women and men, therefore, both give valued elements to the birthing process." Thai men in the North are no exception (cf. Liamputtong, 2000a, b).

The women in this study said their husbands would take care of the newborn, wash nappies, help with household chores, and cook during this period. Even though the women might have their significant others to help, their husbands would still play a key role in providing support. Malai, a poor rural woman, told us that her husband helped her during her confinement period so that she could have good rest and avoid *lom pid duan* for the entire *yu duan* period. Pimjai, a rural poor woman too, said that her husband did all the chores in the house for the first two weeks, as he was afraid that she might be affected by *lom pid duan* if she carried out some tasks, particularly cooking.

Some middle-class women were able to employ a neighbor or a maid to assist them during the *yu duan* period. The helper usually performs all household chores and the preparation of food. This leaves the woman the opportunity for a full rest and to concentrate on taking care of her newborn. For some poor women, however, even though their husbands assisted them during *yu duan*, most could only do it for two weeks or so. The men had to return to work. The women then had to perform household chores and other tasks by themselves if they did not have other significant members to help them. For some poor women, therefore, they might not have a full rest as their middle-class counterparts. This suggests that social support women received varies according to the women's social class background (Oakley, 1988; Oakley & Rajan, 1991).

LOCAL MORAL WORLDS:
PERSISTENCE OR RESISTANCE!

Some observations made by previous social scientists (Muecke, 1976; Mougne, 1978) suggest that the local moral world (Kleinman, 1992) of traditional confinement practice is diminishing in Thailand. The decline of this practice has been suggested that it was due to "a loss of traditions within the context of modernisation" (Whittaker, 2000: 145). However, it appears that the local moral worlds of confinement practices are still prevalent in Chiang Mai today, at least at the time that I conducted this study. This is similar to what Whittaker has recently observed in Northeastern Thailand (2000, 2002).

Although the women in my study gave birth in modern hospitals, they continue to observe *yu duan* practices upon returning home. Women expressed fear of the consequences of not following *yu dual* rituals. This seems to be more prevalent among rural poor women. When the women were asked to articulate their feelings about *yu duan* practices, many would react with a sense of satisfaction. One common remark from the women in this study was that because they observed *yu duan* practices, they did not experience any ill health after giving birth. Even among those who could not elaborate on reasons for the practices, they still believed in the benefit of *yu duan*.

The persistence of *yu duan* practices seems to be more marked with a first birth (cf. Van Gennep, 1966; Whittaker, 2000). For a few urban women, the second birth served as a point of departure from the tradition. They believed that as they had observed the tradition once, it would not be essential with the following birth. Maneeya observed *yu duan* rituals more strictly with her first birth. However, it was mainly due to the influence of her mother who insisted that she must observe *yu duan* rituals. Despite her mother's plea for her to continue to observe *yu duan* rituals, Maneeya did not wish to do so with her second child. She elaborated:

My mother begged me to do it with my second birth. She said even though it was hot I should tolerate it for the benefit of my future health. She said if the body could totally get rid of rotten stuff, when I become older I would not experience aches and pain on my body and when I am exposed to coldness, I would not had cramp. But, I did not believe in so I did not do it. So, mum said "it is up to you, I have warned you but you did not listen to me. Whatever will happen to you then it is your problem." Well, I thought giving birth was already so difficult, why should I torture myself by following the tradition.

The persistence of *yu duan* practice in the local community can be seen from the account of Patanee, an urban educated woman. As she did not strictly observe the *yu duan* ritual, she would carry her newborn with minimum clothes on and walk around the front of her house near the market place. Whenever a passerby saw this, they would make some negative comments on her behaviors.

EMBODYING MODERNITY:
KHON THANSAMAI (BEING MODERN)

Majorie Muecke (1984), Mary Beth Mills (1999), and Andrea Whittaker (2000) point to the pervasive notion of *thansamai* (being modern) discourse among women in Thailand. Mills (1999: 14) suggests, in contemporary Thailand, modernity discourses permeate much of everyday life regardless of people's class backgrounds. These discourses emphasize "images and standards of newness and new time."

Some women in my study embodied divergent worldviews regarding *yu duan* practices in the past (*samai khon*) and the present (*samai ni* or *samai mai*). Middle-class educated women residing in Chiang Mai City embodied modernity to the extent that being modern means a traditional way of life is no longer relevant.

Resistance to traditions seemed to be also prevalent among urban women. Patanee, an urban educated woman, elaborated:

After birth I had to wear a long sleeved top and socks and all sort of things to cover my body. I was a bit stubborn about this. I gave birth in February which was rather hot, so I did not want to follow my mother's advice. So, I was scolded by mum and she said if I didn't do it I would experience aches and pain on my bones when I was a bit older. I said back to her that all older people will have aches and pain on their body anyhow [laugh].

Some educated middle-class women challenged the tradition. Having given birth in a hospital, women had already exposed themselves to activities which were prohibited by tradition. When they were told by family members, they challenged it. For some women, being modern means that tradition has to be modified to some extent. Sinjai, an urban educated woman, also remarked that she only observed certain aspects of *yu duan* practices. For example, she would make her body warm by wearing a hat and socks, but she would not abstain from having a shower as required by the old tradition. Pragmatically, however, for Sinjai, she chose to observe certain traditions, which she believed to be beneficial. This applied to the prohibition of not leaving a room or home in the first thirty days.

Another modification that women mentioned was the binding of the abdomen. Traditionally, a woman may use a piece of long cloth to bind her abdomen to keep it flat. Nowadays, as I have mentioned earlier, women can purchase ready-made underwear known as a "Stay" in modern department stores. Many women used this as it is easy to obtain and it looks more modern and perhaps would be more convenient if the woman wore trousers rather than a sarong as in the old days. This also applies to the use of a ready made piece of rubber for abdominal binding. The rubber band could be easily purchased in stores, and it was believed to be easier to bind the abdomen with. The traditional steam bath has been replaced with a modern sauna used for losing weight. Wasnana, an urban educated woman, for example, went to a house that caters for herbal sauna for losing weight near her home as soon as her *duan* finished.

The modification of postpartum rules seems to be more prevalent among urban middle-class women. Most often women cited inconvenience, lack of time and lack of support as their main reasons for modification. Some mentioned their lack of tolerance as a reason as well. This is particularly so for the intolerance of heat during *yu duan*, and they would use a fan to relieve the heat.

Women's understanding of their bodies also changed due to being modern. Andrea Whittaker (2000) found in her study with women in Isan that "in the past women were more vulnerable to the ill effects of foods after giving birth. Now with modern medicine, birthing in hospital and a more comfortable lifestyle, young women are stronger after birth than older generations." Conversely, some women in this study felt that as they now live in a modern time, their level of tolerance was not the same as older generations.

Some women would observe *yu duan* rituals and follow postpartum restrictions, but might break the rules occasionally. The level of tolerance seems to be reduced with modern life. Orachorn, a poor rural woman, for example admitted that she once or twice turned on a fan during the *yu duan* period, as she could not tolerate the heat. She would turn it off as soon as her mother entered her room. Similarly, she washed her hair twice during this period, as she could not stand the smell of her hair.

As a result of growing up in a modern time, some younger mothers might not follow *yu duan* practices strictly, as they did not have much knowledge about its consequences. Siriporn, an urban educated woman, for example said that she intermittently kept herself warm and avoided going out during *yu duan*, as this was what she was told by older persons.

Notwithstanding, although women mentioned that they did not believe in the old way, they would still observe certain rituals to prevent future ill health. Araya, an urban woman, who did not observe *yu duan* practices, did use warm water for her shower, as her mother informed her that her body was still not in a normal stage and she had fear about some health consequences. She also did not leave home for the whole month after birth. Her reason was that she wanted the wound from a caesarean birth to heal properly, but not because she believed in confining to home as required in the *yu duan* ritual.

MEDICAL INFLUENCES ON TRADITIONAL *YU DUAN* PRACTICES

Western medicine has dominated health and illness behaviors in Thai society since the expansion of Western medicine in Thailand in the 1980s (Sermsri, 1989; see also chapter 1 in this volume). Andrea Whittaker (2000: 57) argues that, since Western biomedicine has been introduced into Thailand, this has "led to the incorporation of a variety of ideas, techniques, and medicines into common usage." In childbirth this is no exception (see chapter 2, 3, and 4 in this volume). Whittaker (2000) also points to the uneasy relationship between modern Western doctors and local villagers in Northeastern Thailand. By giving birth in a hospital, Whittaker (2000: 123) suggests, "women become participants in a process wherein their bodies are constituted as sites of reform and 'modernisation.'" She also suggests that this discourse attempts "to rid village women of what biomedicine defines as 'superstitious beliefs' and 'traditions', and in doing so challenge and alter the subjective meanings of female bodies and the authority of traditional knowledge."

The narratives of women in this study also reveal medical dominance in their thinking and behaviors. Traditionally, women should take as much rest as possible during the *yu duan* period. This meant that they would not walk around. Nowadays, as I have shown in chapters 3 and 4, women give birth in hospitals. They are encouraged by medical professions to walk soon after delivery. Naree, an urban poor woman who gave birth in a teaching hospital in Chiang Mai City, explained:

> In the old days, we would not be allowed to get up and walk around as they were afraid that we might fall and injure ourselves because we would not be strong enough after giving birth. Now, if you are in hospital, they [medical professions] will tell you to walk. The more you walk, the better it will be. Soon after giving birth, they will tell us to walk; we have to even walk to our bed in maternity ward. In hospital, the doctor will tell you to wash your hair, but at home we are not allowed to do so. It is so different.

Foods provided in hospital might not be consumed by women after giving birth as they might be in conflict with traditional diets during *yu duan*. A new mother consumes traditional medicines to flush out remaining childbirth blood and leftover placenta for good health in the future. But, some women would be advised against this by medical practitioner. The consumption of *nam pu leoi* is traditionally promoted, as it assists a proper flow of blood and wind in the body. But, medical professionals discouraged women to do so, as it is believed to cause jaundice and anemia in the mother and a newborn.

However, there were women who would follow medical practitioners' advice for their postpartum practices. Authoritative knowledge of the medical profession (Jordan, 1997; Davis-Floyd & Sargent, 1997; chapter 2) permeates these women's accounts. To these women, their traditions might seem logical but they chose to follow medical advice. Siriporn, an educated urban woman, had this to say about her diet during the confinement period:

I ate everything like beef, chicken, eggs, all of them. I did not have any prescription except for pickle stuff. I followed the booklet given by the hospital about diet and what the hospital staff told me.

Naree, a poor urban woman, remarked that she did not have sexual intercourse for at least one and a half months postpartum due to the advice of her doctor.

We can't have any sex during *yu duan* as our wound is not properly healed and we might be further infected by any infection caused by sexual acts. In the past, it was prohibited by one month but now the doctor would tell us not to have it for at least one and a half months. Some women might have sex soon after their confinement finished and they caught some infections because their wound is not properly healed, so now the doctors would tell you not to do it too soon.

Prapaporn, an urban educated woman, was one of a few mothers in this study who did not observe *yu duan* practices. She commented on many aspects of *yu duan* that she had heard from others, but she chose to follow medical advice. She said, when asked the reason she did not observe *yu duan*, that:

My doctor told me that childbirth is not an illness. It is only the act of giving life to another human being. Giving birth does not make us sick like other sicknesses. So, I believed in it, and I did not do any *yu duan* practices.

CONCLUDING DISCUSSION

Faye Ginsburg and Rayna Rapp (1995: 2) contend that reproduction, including childbirth, is "inextricably bound up with the production of culture."

Childbirth including the period immediately following birth is an event in which traditions are deeply involved (Symonds, 1991). It is seen as "a dangerous and liminal period when a new mother and her newborn are in an 'in-between' world" (Symonds, 1991: 265). As such, the childbirth process is "inherently filled with tension, unpredictability, and danger" (Symonds, 1991: 18). Hence, there are many rules that women and their families must adhere to in order to avoid negative consequences. In this liminal stage, women must be segregated from the society at large (Turner, 1979). As we have seen in this chapter, traditional postpartum beliefs and practices abound in Northern Thailand. However, the level of adherence differs according to the place in the social structure of the women and their families. Poor rural women seem to hold on to their traditions more strongly than their urban counterparts.

As Andrea Whittaker (2000) has pointed out in Northeastern Thailand, the persistence of local moral worlds is also noted markedly in this study. At one level, Whittaker (2000: 140) argues that the persistence of the postpartum care in the local world not only emphasizes the influence and authority of tradition, "but constitutes a form of defence of local practice against the hegemony of Western medical discourse." Postpartum practice continues to survive in Northern Thailand and it is precisely because the practice may be "an important site of the continuance of local identity." This is made possible due to lack of medical surveillance during the postpartum period. As such, the postpartum practice "remains a space in which traditional knowledge remains ascendant" (Whittaker, 2000: 140).

At another level, Whittaker (2000: 146) suggests that the persistence of the postpartum practice "draws attention to the meanings of the practice for the continued fertility of women and is an important aspect of their identity . . . The practice persists owing to its social significance as a rite of passage marking the achievement of mature adult status" (see also Hanks, 1963; Keyes, 1986; Davies, 1994). It seems the women's narratives situate neatly within Whittaker's theoretical explanations.

We also observe the change within the women's accounts. The women's behaviors and practices are changed due to the influence of modernization. Middle-class urban women in particular embody modernity in their thinking and behaviors concerning postpartum practices. As Mary Beth Mills (1999) suggests, poor rural women have not succumbed to modernization to the same extent as urban women and this is mainly due to their marginalized position in the society. But, modernization has brought with it medical dominance. Due to their medical knowledge, doctors retain authoritative knowledge and possess a higher status (Jordan, 1997; Davis-Floyd & Sargent, 1997; chapter 2). The consequence of this dominance is the attempt to dismiss local traditional knowledge and practices.

Despite changes in the women's lives, postpartum beliefs and practices remain an essential part for postpartum care for women and have important consequences for women's health and well-being in Northern Thailand (Boonmongkon et al., 2001, 2002; Whittaker, 2000, 2002; Liamputtong & Naksook, 2003). Many Thai women see their reproductive health problems as the consequence of inadequate postpartum practices (Boonmongkon et al., 2001, 2002; Whittaker, 2000, 2002; Liamputtong & Naksook, 2003). Thai women also believed that the effects of postpartum taboos would continue for the rest of their lives. It is imperative that postpartum care for women incorporates local traditions so that women's health can be optimized at the time when they are in the most vulnerable stage of their lives.

Chapter Six

Becoming a Mother

How do you feel about becoming a mother?

I immediately think of my own mother. . . . I love my baby so deeply that I can't find a word to express my feeling and this makes me think that my mother must have felt like this when she had me. When I was young I didn't think that my mother loved me that much. But, once I become a mother I realize how much she had loved me. And, this makes me feel even closer to my mother. (Naree)

INTRODUCTION

Research concerning motherhood in the past decade has taken a social constructionist or feminist standpoint (Oakley, 1980; Boulton, 1983; Wearing, 1984; Ussher, 1990; Phoenix & Woollett, 1991; Richardson, 1993; Brown et al., 1994; Ribbens, 1994; Brown et al., 1997; Weaver & Ussher, 1997). An interesting pattern emerging from these studies is that motherhood is seen "as an area of ambivalence for women" (Weaver & Ussher, 1997: 51; Oakley, 1980; Wearing, 1984; DiQuinzio, 1999; Manne, 2005). Mary Boulton (1983), for example, interviewed mothers from middle- and working-class backgrounds about motherhood and daily lives. Women in her study expressed contradiction with their feelings of being a mother. Motherhood was burdensome, but it also provided enjoyment and pleasure. Despite negative aspects of motherhood, women described motherhood as rewarding. Similar patterns have also been found in Stephanie Brown and others' study (1994) with Australian-born women in Melbourne.

Recently, Jane Weaver and Jane Ussher (1997: 51) examined the expectations, experiences, and motherhood changes among mothers of young children in North London. Similarly, they found that "societal myths were implicated for giving a false impression of motherhood." When this is combined with the high demands of child care, it led to "disillusionment and a sense of lost identity." The reality of being a mother is contrary to the idealized image of motherhood normally presented in the media to society. This made many women feel inadequate. Some women found that they were seen as "just a mother," implying that motherhood is a normal mundane part of womanhood and mothers are people without intelligence and status. This reinforces the image of "lost self" (64) among women in this study. Despite this image, women tried to find ways which they can use to counteract negative aspects of motherhood by emphasizing the positive emotional aspects of motherhood and affirming to themselves that even though their lives were changed after becoming a mother, their inner selves were not affected by motherhood. Women also pointed to the positive side of motherhood, particularly the joys of seeing their child grow and their deep emotional warmth and love for their child.

At present, the study of motherhood among Thai women is largely non-existent. Those who have written on Thai women and childbearing concentrated on childbirth experiences and customs (Hanks, 1963; Anuman Rajadhon, 1987; Mougne, 1978; Muecke, 1976; Poulsen, 1983; Whittaker, 1995; Liamputtong Rice & Naksook, 1998a, 1998b; Naksook & Liamputtong Rice, 1999; Liamputtong Rice et al., 1999) or the lived experience of motherhood of Thai immigrant women (Liamputtong, 2001; Liamputtong & Naksook, 2003a, b), and Southeast Asian including Lao, Cambodian, and Vietnamese women (Liamputtong, 2006) living in Australia. In this chapter, the experiences of Northern Thai women will be used as a paradigm case to discuss the meanings and experiences of motherhood in the current social, cultural, and economical context of Northern Thai society. In the chapter, I first examine women's discourses of the meanings of motherhood. I then look at their lived experiences of being a mother and their perceptions of health associated with motherhood. The chapter also looks at mothering and women's relationships with their husbands and other family members.

MOTHERHOOD AS A "MORAL CAREER"

In this chapter, I situate my discussions within Erving Goffman's (1963) theoretical framework of "moral career": women and a moral career of motherhood. Career, according to Goffman (1961: 119), refers to "any social strand of any person's course through life." Goffman (1961: 119) argues that "such a career is not a thing that can be brilliant or disappointing; it can no more be a success than a failure." I contend that Goffman's concept is a useful framework for the understanding of women's moral career as mothers. As Goffman (1961: 119) puts it, the framework provides a "two-sidedness" which links internal matters such as the image of self and self-identity (the image of self and self-identity as mothers) with broader structures that include the "publicly accessible institutional complex" (the institution of motherhood). As such, Goffman's notion of career enables an individual to "move back and forth" between individual agency and social structure; that is between "the self and its significant society" (1961: 119). According to Maria Zadoroznyj (1999: 273), the centrality of Goffman's argument is its emphasis on the temporality of the development of "self" in a "career." Therefore, this involves the important process of the "labeled" developing an identity interacting with others with the power to "label." In this sense, women may develop self-identity as mothers and be labeled as good or bad mothers as they interact with others around them.

Goffman refers "moral" to "self-conceptions" or "the experience of the self" (McMahon, 1995). Goffman (1963: 45) suggests that individuals who have "similar changes in conceptions of self" share "moral career," which in turn may be "both cause and effect of commitment to a similar sequence of personal adjustments." As such, the women in my study share similar changes in self-perceptions of being a mother, hence motherhood becomes a "moral career" for women who mother their children. Following arguments made by Nancy Chodorow (1978) and Carol Gilligan (1982), Martha McMahon (1995) suggests that through motherhood, women achieve the moral characteristic of giving and caring. In this chapter, I also refer to moral career of mothers as not only changes in their self-perceptions, but also changes that occur in relation with the ethics of care and responsibility of women (Chodorow, 1978; McMahon, 1995).

Goffman's conceptual framework of "moral career" is related to the concept of "identity." Identity, according to symbolic interactionists, is formed through shared social interaction. People make sense of their experiences through a common set of symbols and these symbols are developed and find meaning through an interaction (Strauss, 1959; Blumer, 1969; Brubaker & Cooper, 2000). Following Pierre Bourdieu (1977), Rogers Brubaker and Frederick Cooper (2000: 4) suggest that identity is conceptualized as a "category of practice." Identity, as a category of practice, is "used by 'lay' actors in some everyday settings to make sense of themselves, of their activities, of what they share with, and how they differ from, others." In the case of Thai mothers I discuss in this chapter, I suggest that identity as the category of practice is adopted by the women to make sense of themselves as mothers and their mothering roles.

BECOMING A MOTHER

Becoming a mother has several meanings among Thai women in this study. The following themes represent women's discourses about being a mother.

Happiness and Pride

To many women, becoming a mother gave them happiness and pride (cf. McMahon, 1995; Brown et al., 1997; Liamputtong, 2006). They felt happy because they were able to fulfill the role of womanhood as is expected in the Thai cultural context (Liamputtong & Naksook, 2003b). They were proud because they had brought another life into this world. The happiness and pride were more marked when the child they produced was physically and mentally normal and when they could see that the way they mothered would make the child grow up to be a good person. Saijai, an urban woman, remarked:

> I feel so glad and proud of becoming someone's mother. Because when you have children you have the opportunity to teach and train your children. When your children turn up to be a good person you feel so glad and happy. When your children are not naughty and they help you, you feel so glad. This is what it is like, to be a mother, isn't it!

Becoming a mother, in the women's eyes, also meant security in old age as they believed there would be someone to take care of them when they would no longer be able to perform duties and earn their living (see chapter 1 in this volume).

> I am glad that I have become a mother. I am happy that now I have got children. When I see their faces, it makes me so happy and cheerful. I am also happy that there will be someone looking after me when I am old. (Srinang, a rural poor woman)

Bringing up children, the women said, was tiring since they had to take responsibility for other tasks as well as child care (see chapter 8 in this volume). This was particularly so when they had no one to assist them. Despite the exhaustion, when they saw their children's faces or when the children showed affection towards them, this made them happy and they valued motherhood greatly.

> I am proud of becoming a mother. Becoming a mother makes me happy. Sometimes I feel frustrated because I have too many things to do. I have to do everything without help. This makes me very tired. But, when the children call me "*mae*" [mother] and give me a hug or a kiss, I just feel so happy and forget all the hard work. (Ruchira, a rural woman)

But, children also brought joy and other positive aspects to their life despite hard work in raising them. In times of problems, the presence of children was most valued. They believed that only children could help them to go through tough times in their lives. Daranee, an urban woman, contended:

> Having children of your own can help you a great deal. This is particularly when you are not happy or when you have troubles in your life. When you see your children they provide you with emotional support in order to fight with difficulties.

Self-Sacrifice and Endless Concern

For most women, once they became a mother, the children would come first for everything (Brown et al., 1994; Liamputtong, 2006; Rendina & Liamputtong, 2006). Saijai, an urban educated woman, remarked:

> When you become a mother you have to sacrifice everything for your children, everything. Like you will not spend money on yourself but on your children. Before you buy a piece of cloth, you would think about your children. Then, you would not buy it. You have to keep the money for your children. Whatever you do, you think about your children first.

Becoming a mother would make them endlessly worried and concerned about their children (see also chapter 8).

> My feelings change a lot after I become a mother. Whatever I do, I am always worried about my children and I have to think about my children first. I can't just indulge myself and go off to do whatever I want to as I used to be. The children always come first. (Sira, an urban woman)

Another feature in this theme expressed by the women is that of endurance. Once becoming a mother, one must be able to endure the difficult situations which might come into their lives. Women believed that if they were not able to endure life themselves, they would not be able to take care and protect their children properly.

> When you have become a mother you must endure everything; whether it is something about your children or any other household matters. Whatever comes into your life, you must endure greatly. (Daranee, an urban woman)

Responsibility and Maturity

Women expressed that their lives had changed dramatically as a result of becoming a mother (McMahon, 1995; Liamputtong, 2006). Becoming a mother made them more responsible for everything, but particularly for their children.

> Becoming a mother makes me more responsible than before. When I was by myself, I did whatever I wanted to. But, now whatever I do, I think about my children first. It is like there is something I have to take responsibility for all the time. (Sira, an urban woman)

Responsibility seems to run parallel to the perception of self-sacrifice (cf. Ribbens et al., 2000; Barnard, 2005; Liamputtong, 2006). Women would prepare to stop everything for their own child, as Wasana, an urban educated woman, suggested:

> My life changed a lot after I become a mother. It changes in a way of my responsibility. I take more responsibility for my baby. If he is not well I cannot stay at work. I just have to go to pick him up from school and stay home with him. I can neglect my work when it comes to the health of my child. I have to choose my child first.

Being a mother, in their views, also helped one to become more mature because one must learn how to take responsibility and control one's emotion and behavior.

> I feel that I am maturer since I become a mother. Before, I always acted childishly. But, since becoming a mother I think more like an adult. Whatever I do, I must think first. Before, I always argued with my husband even for a minor matter. Like when he went out just for a short while I would complain about it. But, since I have the baby, I don't care. He can do whatever he wants to. (Payao, a rural woman)

Not only does one have to take more responsibility for one's children, women also believed that they must take more responsibility for their own lives and well-being. This was to ensure they would live long enough to take care of their children. Women were anxious about leaving their children as orphans. Who would look after the children if they no longer lived was the question women frequently asked themselves. This prompted them to be more cautious about their own well-being.

> Becoming a mother makes me more careful with myself. I have to be more careful because I have to take care of my kids. Whatever I do I think about my kids first. What I fear most in my life now is to die when my children are still young. It is like I have to leave them under the care of other people. And, my kids will not have parents to take care of them. (Patanee, an urban woman)

Appreciation of Love and *Bun Khun* (Gratitude) of One's Own Mother

All women made the statement about their own mothers when talking about becoming a mother. Being a mother provided them with a feeling which was not easy to express or explain. It was, however, the best feeling they had ever had in their lifetime. This feeling made them realize how much love they had received from their own mothers.

> It is the best feeling that I have ever had. It is the feeling that only a mother can feel. You will not appreciate this feeling if you have not been a mother. When you have become a mother that feeling tells you how much your mother loves you. . . . The love you have from your mother will be transmitted to your baby when you are a mother. (Suriya, a rural poor woman)

Sira, an urban woman, expressing her feelings about becoming a mother reflected on what her own mother's feelings might have been when she was a young child, and nearly shed tears in the interview when she said:

> After I have my kids I always think about my mother. I shed tear many times because I realize how difficult it was for her to bring me up. I also understand deeply about my mother's feelings toward motherhood. Before I have my kids, I didn't think much about it, but when I have my own kids, I know exactly how my mother felt when she had me.

Women said that childbirth helped them to realize the hard work involved in giving birth and that of bringing children up. This made them love their own mothers more. As Areeya, an urban educated woman, put it this way:

> I feel happy that I have given a life to another human being and it makes me think about my mother more. It makes me realized that my mother is so brave because she has five children and how exhausted she would be. I have only two children and I feel so exhausted already. It makes me love my mother more because I think my mother would probably love me the way I love my children.

Women admitted that when they were younger they did not really listen to their mothers' advice. However, when they had become a mother and when they did not know how to handle things with child care and childrearing, they always thought about their mothers. This prompted them to listen to their mothers more.

Most often, however, women mentioned that becoming a mother made them appreciate the *bun khun* of their mothers more. *Bun khun* in the Thai context refers to gratitude toward the love and kindness of one's mother in giving birth and bringing them up (see chapter 1 in this volume).

> Becoming a mother is just like what old persons always say that if you are a woman you will know your mother's *bun khun* when you become a mother. When you have to cope with difficulties in bringing up your own children, it will make you realize how difficult it was for your own mother in bringing you up too. We would really appreciate our mothers' *bun khun* when we have become a mother. (Srinang, a rural poor woman)

Becoming a mother and realizing how much love and care one's own mother had for them made the women realize that they must take more care of their mothers. This belief tended to come from those who believed that they had not really looked after their mothers well in the past. Prapaporn, an urban woman elaborated:

> After becoming a mother I realize how good my mother is and it makes me love my mother more. I also feel sorry for my mother too, so I look after her much better than before. When I was younger, I did not really listen to my mother. I always argued with her. But, when I become a mother, I feel that I have to pay back her *bun khun*. I have to do it when she is still alive. If you don't do it now and if she passes away, then it will be too late to pay back her *bun khun*. Now, I look after her very well; I do my best to take good care of her. This is the way I pay back her *bun khun*.

One woman, interestingly, contended that becoming a mother changed her relationship with her father. When she was younger, she said, she did not like her father and always had arguments with him when he drank too much. But, when she had a child, her husband helped her a great deal in caring for the baby. His caring nature made her realized that her own father might have done a similar thing to her when she was an infant. This prompted her to contact her father, and since then, their relationship had improved.

MOTHERHOOD AND HEALTH

Women were asked to compare their health prior to and after giving birth. Most women believed that their health had changed to some extent (cf. Macintyre & Dennerstein, 1995; Liamputtong & Naksook, 2003a; Liamputtong, 2006). However, the perceived causes varied. Some said that the change was due to their age.

> After I have two children I started to feel aches and pains on my body. First it started with pains on my knees and now I have cramps very often. I think be-

cause I am getting older. When one gets older, one always feels pains on arms and legs and so on anyhow. (Srinang, a rural poor woman)

Others said that childbearing had depleted their energy and health. Becoming pregnant and having to nourish the baby in their body for nine months as well as giving birth and losing blood from the body were seen to make them weaker. Patanee, an urban woman, elaborated:

I feel that I am now not that healthy as before I have the baby. Before, I hardly became ill. Occasionally, I would feel a bit sick. But, now I feel that I tend to get sick easily, things like a common cold and backache. I think having children is just like we have to use all strength in our body. For example, when the baby is in our body we have to use good things in our body to nourish the baby. So, after we give birth, it makes our body weak. Giving birth too makes us weak, I believe.

Exhaustion and hard work of raising a child are seen as a main cause of their ill health. Payao, a rural poor woman, had this to say:

After I have the baby, I loss weight and even now I still loss weight. I think because I do not have enough sleep and do not eat properly. When I want to get something to eat and the baby cries, someone would scold me to attend to my children. Also, I think because the baby is taking my [breast] milk; she is taking my blood away from my body. This is why my health is now not as good as before.

Many women, however, believed that their worse health was due to the fact that they did not observe traditional confinement practices properly. During a period of thirty days after birth, Northern Thai women traditionally follow the confinement practice called *yu duan* (see chapter 5 in this volume). The practice is to prevent a new mother having contact with wind which is seen as dangerous since the wind, once it enters the body, can cause all sorts of health problems including headache, shivering, fever, and being susceptible to the change of weather. These ill symptoms are referred generally as *pid duan* or *lom pid duan*. It is commonly believed that this condition cannot be cured. Once a woman has it, it will recur throughout her lifetime. Many women were particularly cautious about their confinement practices, but some might not observe the practice strictly, particularly when they did not believe in the old way.

When I was younger I hardly had any cold and flu. But, after I have a child I got cold and flu very easily. And now, I feel the cold very easily. Even in summer when we turn on the air conditioner, I will feel very cold whereas my husband does not feel it. I have to cover myself with blankets. My husband says that may be it is *pid duan*. When I was *yu duan*, I only wore socks which covered my ankles, not the whole legs. People told me to wear socks covering high up on my legs, like a soccer player does. But, I did not want to do that; it looked ugly on my legs. I also did not wear a thick top, just a thin material one. My husband thinks that it is because of *pid duan*, and I think it may be that too. Why didn't I have this problem before I had my baby! (Siriporn, an urban woman)

Women who come from poor families tended to attribute their poor health after giving birth to lack of the opportunity to follow Thai traditional confinement practices fully. This was mainly due to a lack of familial support for them to rest and follow *yu duan* as well as a lack of opportunity to consume proper confinement food. This is what Wasana, an urban poor woman, told us:

My health changes a lot after I have had children. This is particularly when the weather is cold. I will feel the cold more than anyone. When I have a cold shower, I will shiver. It is really cold into my body. Now I have to take only a warm shower, I can't have a cold shower even it is in the summer. I think because after having a few children my health deteriorates because I did not follow *yu duan* fully and I did not eat confinement food properly. I can't do that because no one helps me and I am too poor to get someone to help me.

Some women who experienced worse health after childbirth had tried to regain their health by resorting to self-help approaches including limiting drinks to only warm water and having a regular herbal steam sauna. These approaches would help to get rid of "poison" in their body.

I drink only warm water in the morning and afternoon every day. I also go to a place where I can have herbal steam sauna to steam my body. They put some herbs including tamarind, turmeric and honey in it to steam my body. This will make my body strong again since it will get rid of poisonous stuff [from childbirth] from my body and it will make my skin look good too. I do this once a week and I have been doing it for a while now. I feel much better now. I feel comfortable in the body since I no longer feel heavy in the body, but I still feel tired. (Wasana, an urban poor woman)

Nevertheless, there were also women who believed that their health was much better after they had a baby (cf. Liamputtong & Naksook, 2003a; Liamputtong, 2006). This was because of the demand of motherhood which required them to move about and perform many tasks in looking after the children. These movements or activities were seen as a form of exercise which helped them to become stronger. In addition, they must also keep themselves fit and strong, otherwise who would take care of the children. Nida, an urban poor woman, said:

After I had my baby my health improved a lot because I looked after him and this was the same as doing exercise. Besides, I cannot afford to be weak. I must be strong. If I am weak or sick, who would look after my baby!

Those who said that their health did not change after having children believe that it is due to the fact that they observed traditional practices strictly.

> Before I had my children I was healthy and it is still the same after I have had two kids. I think because I did not eat anything wrong when I was in confinement. I did *yu duan* as what old people told me to do so. Whatever they told me not to do, I did not do it. (Isara, a rural poor woman)

Despite the fact that they followed traditional practices during the confinement period, women continued to restrict themselves even long after childbirth in order to prevent ill health in the future. They believe that childbirth changed their bodies to some extent. The loss of bodily nourishment during pregnancy and blood during birth made their bodies less immune to illnesses and diseases (cf. Liamputtong & Naksook, 2003a). To protect their vulnerable bodies, women were cautious about their food and behaviours. Manee, a rural woman, told us:

> I believe that being able to follow traditional confinement practices helps to maintain my good health a lot. Even nowadays, I am still being careful with what I do. If there is a bad smell somewhere, I would escape from it. Even though I no longer do *yu duan*, I still have to look after my body because after childbirth your body changes. It is like you have a personal illness. *Roke pid duan* can appear at any time of your life because your body has lost blood and water from giving birth. And, this makes your body less immune to illnesses.

Some also said that their health improved after giving birth and they attributed this to the fact that they observed traditional confinement practices strictly.

> Old people always tell you that you have to observe the confinement practices so that your health will be maintained after we give birth to our children. I followed their advice strictly and I think it contributes to my good health now too. My health still very good after I give birth! It is even better than before too. (Naree, an urban poor woman)

SUPPORTS AND CONFLICTS WITH FAMILY MEMBERS

Most women had familial support due to the nature of extended family in northern Thailand. The women lived with their husbands and their own natal families. Only a few women lived with their parents-in-law. When needed, women always received support. This was particularly so during the confinement period when they needed good rest for recovery. However, when it came to rearing children, there were some tensions and conflicts. Very often, women said that grandparents tended to spoil their children, and they believed this would not be good for the children.

> I think that the kids should not be too spoiled and I want everyone in the family to treat the kids like that. But, my parents really spoil my kids, especially my father. They just do whatever my kids want to do. I told them not to spoil the kids, but they do not agree. So, we have an argument. There are some conflicts like this in our family. (Patanee, an urban woman)

Some mothers wished to look after their children their own way, but this could be in contrary to what the family did. This created frustration among the women. Warunee, an urban woman, elaborated:

> Very often I have conflicts with my parents-in-law. For example, I prepare a solid food according to a manual or a book. But, my mother-in-law says that I should just feed my child anything so that when he is older he can eat anything. If I follow the book, the child does not grow up properly. When the baby was not well, I wanted to take him to a doctor, but my in-laws would say that just give him some medicines because he was not really sick and why should I spend money on doctors. But, he is my child and if something happened to him I would be very sorry. So, I took him to see a doctor. I just ignored them. Another thing is taking care of my child. When I did not work, I did everything. But, now I am working and I want my husband to share the task of taking care of my baby. My in-laws do not approve of this. They say I should look after him myself, not their son. But, I am also working; why can't he help me?

Most women also had some conflict with their husbands in bringing up their children; however it was not to the same extent as the conflicts with their parents or parents-in-law. Most often these were merely minor conflicts which they believed could occur in any family. These conflicts included the way they treated their children. Some mothers were blamed for indulging their children and vice versa for their husbands.

> I tend to pay too much attention to my children and do everything for them because I love them so much. But, my husband would tell me that I should not do that. I should leave the children to look after themselves too; don't do everything for them because I would spoil them. Spoiled children are not good children. He wants my children to be good like other people's children. So, he does not want me to do everything for my children. (Sinjai, an urban woman)

Some said that they were accused of being too self-centered, thinking only about their own needs, not those of the child's and this created tension and conflict with their husbands. Others said that tension and conflict occurred when they scolded or hit their children in time of anger.

A conflict with my husband, yes of course it does occur sometimes. When the kid is so naughty and does not listen to me when I try to teach him, it makes me angry and I would hit him. Then my husband would be angry with me because he thinks that it is only a minor matter I don't have to hit the kid, just talk to him. And when I try to teach him what should be done or what should not be done, he would be angry too because he thinks I talk too much. (Sangchan, a rural woman)

Women remarked that they were also judged on their performance as mothers from their husbands as well as their mothers-in-law. Most often they were criticized for not being a good enough mother, as Manee, a rural woman, elaborated:

Sometimes when the baby's asleep I would walk over to my next door friend and talk with her. At one time, I carried on with the conversation and forgot about the baby. When the baby awoke, he cried because I was not there. My husband called me back to get the baby, but I did not hear him, so he scolded me that I am not a good mother. Also, I am a good sleeper and when the baby wakes up at night, I tend not to hear him. Once the baby cried because he wet himself and I did not get up to change his nappy. My mother-in-law had to get up and change the nappy, and she scolded me again that I am not a good mother.

Some women believed they had no difficulties in bringing up their children with their husbands since they gave their husbands freedom with childrearing and child care. Women said that even though what their husbands did was not really what they wished, they tended to ignore the behavior. This would create harmony in the family. In addition, women also believed that their husbands left childrearing matters to them, as is the Thai custom for a mother to take this responsibility. Their husbands, therefore, did not interfere with their childrearing practices.

With rearing our kids, my husband leaves it to me. I think because he is a Northern Thai man he is not interested in looking after children. He thinks it is the responsibility of a woman. So, he leaves everything to me and we don't have any conflicts about rearing our kids. (Laksan, a rural woman)

For some women, their husbands also became maturer and felt more responsible for the family. Sira, an urban woman, said:

Since we have the baby, my relationship with my husband has improved greatly. He becomes more mature too. Before we had the baby, he would go out with his friends and get drunk. He did not come home until 8 or 9 o'clock at night and he also gambled when he had money. Since we have the baby, he just works to earn money and looks after the baby.

Others said their husbands helped them with childrearing and housework since they realized that looking after young children was exhausting. Some women even said that their husbands took care of their children more than themselves.

> I don't have conflicts with my husband because we help each other in looking after him. When you have a child, you must help each other. If he does not help, we would probably have lot of arguments. Looking after a child alone is so exhausting. My husband loves taking care of my child more than me. When he comes home from work, he can see that I am very tired from taking care of the baby all day, so he helps me. (Suriya, a rural woman)

CONCLUDING DISCUSSION

In this chapter, I have shown that many of the lived experiences of Thai women in my study are similar to those of mainstream, Western women in literature, but there are many aspects too that set them apart from their Western counterparts. It is clear that the women in this study felt a profound change through the process of becoming a mother; as in Martha McMahon's term (1995) they experience the "transformation of self." Motherhood, McMahon (1995: 158) suggests, plays "a symbolic role in integrating issues of individual identity, moral choice, and social commitment in the women's lives." Nancy Chodorow (1978: 6) too contends that motherhood "stands out in its emotional and intensity and meaning, and it its centrality for women's lives and social definition." This is clearly seen in the discourses of the women who took part in this study.

Becoming a mother was experienced as a moral transformation of self and women were urged to perform their moral careers. A mother has a moral career; she is a gatekeeper of morality. To be a moral mother, one needs to follow the rules of motherhood knowingly (Murphy, 1999). These rules are "expressive of the extent to which the social worth of motherhood and mothers is currently contested" in the society in which these women live (McMahon, 1995: 190). It is not too surprising to see the women in this study enlisted prescriptions of moral mothers in so many ways.

According to Nancy Chodorow (1978) and Carol Gilligan (1982), women's moral career is influenced by an ethics of care and responsibility for others. Motherhood, Martha McMahon (1995: 274) argues, permits women to obtain "a loving, caring and responsible" feminine identity. In addition, being responsible for their children is about "being moral as a person." As such, motherhood is associated with "female morality." Then motherhood has "high personal value and moral worth" (McMahon 1995: 271). Gilligan (1982) also suggests that women's perception of care and responsibility is seen through their connectedness with others. Becoming a mother, according to Barbara Katz Rothman (1989: 60-63), is "the physical embodiment of connectedness." As McMahon (1995) has suggested in her study, the importance of connectedness with, and responsibility for, others was prevalent in women's ways of thinking. This, too, was expressed by the women in my study. In McMahon's study (1995), she found that through connectedness and responsibility for their children, motherhood brings forth an adult identity. However, for the women in this study, women's connectedness with "others" extended beyond their children. They not only talked about their connectedness with their children, but women also connected to "social others" such as their mothers.

As Ann Phoenix and Anne Woollett (1991) argue, the meanings of motherhood are multi-faceted, Thai women in this study too see motherhood in a variety of ways. Common to all women is the perception that motherhood is not an easy task; endless child care and energy put into mothering is continuous and tiring. Some women believe that motherhood means self-sacrifice and endless concern. But, others believe that motherhood brings joy and pleasure to their lives. This overpowering sense of love and involvement with the child made the negative aspects worthwhile (Boulton, 1983; Weaver & Ussher, 1997). In their study, Jane Weaver and Jane Ussher (1997: 65) also found that the discourses around the theme of overwhelming love highlight "the positive emotional aspects of motherhood."

Previous research undertaken with Western women tends to, or at least partially, interpret motherhood as a negative aspect of women's lives (Antonis, 1981; Ussher, 1990; Phoenix & Woollett, 1991; Woollett & Phoenix, 1991; Weaver & Ussher, 1997; Brown et al., 1997; DiQuinzio, 1999). Weaver and Ussher (1997: 59) for example point out in their study that women see motherhood as mandatory and women must not be selfish by putting themselves before their children. Because of this belief, many women feel frustrated and at times motherhood has "led to a feeling of hopelessness." This pattern is not observed in my study. Although women see their role as "a selfless Madonna" who is prepared to sacrifice everything for their children, motherhood does not contain the negative image as presented in Weaver and Ussher's study (1997).

Weaver and Ussher (1997) suggest hat the most overwhelming part of becoming a mother is the change that it brings to a woman's life, particularly to her perception of herself. As suggested by Goffman (1961, 1963), women have a moral career to perform. This is also true with the women in my study. However, changes tend to be positive. These include motherhood making them to be more responsible toward everything including their own well-being and it makes themselves and their spouses more mature. This is, however, not to say that there are no negative aspects of motherhood among Thai women in this study. Women mention several negative perspectives including putting the child before themselves and the continuation of worry and concern about the well-being and health of their child. Motherhood, to some women, also means worse health for them (Liamputtong & Naksook, 2003a; Liamputtong, 2006).

That the level of low satisfaction with motherhood and its consequent unhappiness found in several studies with women from Western societies which does not exist in this study is interesting. One may speculate on this and conclude that the societal expectation of motherhood in Thai culture and family support women received when they become mothers is of emotional benefit to women. As I have pointed out in chapter 1, in the Thai society in general, and in a "female-centred" system (Potter, 1977: 20) observed in Northern Thailand in particular, motherhood is seen as an ability to bring a new life into the matrilineal line of the family. Girls will strengthen the matriliny of their mothers. Boys, once married, will contribute to the continuity of their wives' matrilineal line. Hence, children are highly valued in Thai society. A woman is, therefore, encouraged to become pregnant as soon as possible after marriage. After giving birth, she is looked after well by the family members so that she can rest to regain her health after a long period of pregnancy and birth (see chapter 5). This is a reward for her for producing a child to ensure the continuity of her matrilineal line. These beliefs and practices, thus, serve to assist a new mother to cope with the demand of motherhood. This helps women to see motherhood as a positive aspect of their lives; in contrast to the viewpoint of being oppressed by the social system of many women in Western societies (McMahon, 1995).

Family members including their spouses and others play a significant role in the way women become a mother and mother their children. This also affects their perceptions of motherhood too. Most women in this study, particularly all those who live in Mae Chantra sub-district, live with their extended families. The support they receive during the postpartum period and thereafter helps them to cope with the demands of child care. As mentioned, for the whole month after giving birth women are required to rest. All household chores including taking care of a newborn infant are undertaken by other family members, particularly their mothers and sisters and in many cases, even their fathers. They are "other mothers" who provide support to mothers. Husbands also play a significant role in this. The support women receive helps them not to feel isolated, as they are surrounded by their kin. This is contrary to the findings of previous studies. Sue Sharpe (1984), for example, points to the isolation women experience because they spend a large amount of time at home with their young children. In Jane Weaver and Jane Ussher's study (1997) women felt tied to the house with their children. In Stephanie Brown and others' study (1997), they also comment that isolation is real for many Australian-born women. This is largely, perhaps, because women in these studies do not have "other mothers" whom they can rely on in bringing up their young children. These two reasons help to explain why Thai women's perceptions and experiences of motherhood are different from their Western counterparts.

A noticeable pattern among the women in this study is the fact that they see their relationship with their own mothers as a very important aspect of becoming a mother. Often, women would mention their own mothers as the first response to my question of what it is like when one becomes a mother. This reflects strong female ties among Thai women, as discussed in chapter 1. Kalwant Bhopal (1998) has also found similar, however to a lesser extent, ties among South Asian women in London. This relationship is, interestingly, absent among research reported among women from Anglo-Celtic backgrounds.

One aspect of Thai cultural beliefs and practices emerging from this study is the notion of *bun khun* of their own mothers expressed by the women. As I have suggested in chapter 1, *bun khun* is a common and pervasive belief among the Thais regardless of gender, class, educational, and regional backgrounds. Similar reflections are found among women in my study when referring to their own mothers.

Women's perceptions of their own health after becoming a mother also present a remarkable pattern. Here again, we see a variety of responses from the women. Although women believe that their health becomes worse, the causes of their health status are multi-faceted. Some see this as due to their age. Others believe that childbirth depletes their strength and energy. What is interesting is the belief that it is due to not following Thai traditional confinement practices. This is confirmed by the belief given by women that their health is maintained after giving birth to one or two children because they follow traditional practices strictly.

It is clear that becoming a mother and to mother well are no easy tasks. A common response from women about becoming a mother is similar to the following statement made by one woman: "Being a mother is not easy. Before I had my child I thought being a mother is an easy thing to do, but it is not so." Hence, what seems to be a societal expectation that, motherhood is an instinctive part of womanhood and mothering is easy, are not true with how the women in my study see it. It confirms that motherhood is a very complex matter indeed.

Chapter Seven

Breast is Best?
Infant Feeding in a
Changing Social Context

ϰ

The practice of breastfeeding has been a key to the survival of the human species and a symbol of motherhood. Although viewed by many health professionals and the public as a benign lifestyle choice, it is a contentious issue, laden with conflicting social, moral and biomedical connotations.

(Guttman, & Zimmerman, 2000: 1457)

INTRODUCTION

Breastfeeding is profoundly supported by both professionals and lay individuals (Schmied & Lupton, 2001: Cricco-Lizza, 2004, 2005). It is claimed that breastfeeding is beneficial for both a newborn infant and a mother (Lawrence, 1995; Newman, 1995; Van Esterik & Menon, 1996; American Academy of Pediatrics, 1997; Enger et al., 1997; Coates & Riordan, 2005). For the infant, breast milk is "the ideal food in both quantity and quality" (Wilmoth & Elder, 1995:579). With its anti-infective properties, breast milk provides protection against infection (Gerrard, 1974; Weller & Dungy, 1986). Breastfeeding also provides bonding between mother and her infant (Jelliffe & Jelliffe, 1978; Howell et al., 1986; Dettwyler, 1995). Hence, breastfeeding is seen as promoting not only the health of the infant, but also its development and psychological well-being (Walker, 1993; Lawrence, 1995; Riordan, 1997; Abel et al., 2001). For the mother, breastfeeding soon after birth reduces the risk of postpartum hemorrhage (Gonzalez, 1990). In addition, it provides a natural form of birth spacing (Brown, 1982; Gray et al., 1990). Economically, breastfeeding saves money which the family has to spend on expensive formula if bottle-feeding is adopted (Jelliffe & Jelliffe, 1978; Wilmoth & Elder, 1995; Abel et al., 2001).

However, not all women and their families necessarily perceive it as such. Infant feeding practices occur within the social and cultural context of the society in which women live (Manderson, 1982; Liamputtong, 2002; Dykes, 2005). Although women understand the value of breast milk, many women choose not to breastfeed their infants or may try to combine breastfeeding with bottle-feeding (Matich & Sims, 1992; Earle, 2000; Dykes, 2005). Previous studies have identified the many reasons women cite as the choice of infant feeding, for example, work (Nardi, 1985; Wright et al., 1993; Yimyam, 1997, Yimyam et al., 1999), insufficient milk (Gussler & Briesemeister, 1980; Greiner et al., 1981; Tully & Dewey, 1985; Winikoff et al., 1988; Hillervik-Lindquist, 1991; Liamputtong, 2002; Moffat, 2002), infant and maternal health (Rossiter, 1992, 1994), lack of social support (Raphael, 1975; Hung et al., 1985; Matich & Sims, 1992; Bailey et al., 2004; Ingram & Johnson, 2004), and availability of infant formula (Jelliffe & Jelliffe, 1978; Van Esterik, 1985; Liamputtong, 2002).

In the several past decades, rapid social and economic transformations have changed women's lives in many parts of the world, and Thai women have also been caught in this change. As I have suggested in chapter 1, women in Thailand have entered the labor force as a way to increase their family income since the 1960s when the country's economy has become increasingly dependent on the global market economy. Many women in the North, as Susanha Yimyam (1997: iv) points out, "work outside the home as well as perform housework . . . Labour force participation for women in the childbearing years has increased rapidly, particularly in the non-agricultural sector." These changes, Yimyam (1997) contends, have profoundly affected women, motherhood, and infant feeding practices (see also Tantiwiramanond & Pandey 1991; Boonyoen et al., 1998; Yimyam & Morrow, 2003).

Similar to many other developing countries, the duration of breastfeeding declined in Thailand during the 1970s (Knodel et al., 1990). Although the decline was moderate, it was pervasive enough to affect women from rural and urban settings as well as women from different educational attainments. How would mothers in Thailand see themselves as mothers and practice infant feeding in a changing social and economic environment? If women have to work outside their homes and try to breastfeed at the same time, will this impact their perceptions and practices of infant feeding? What is the impact of recent economic turmoil in Thailand on motherhood and infant feeding practices?

In this chapter, I discuss infant feeding practices in Northern Thai society. In particular, I focus on how mothers perceive and experience breastfeeding and how they feed their infants. I shall also show the way these mothers interact with health-care professionals with regard to infant feeding attempts.

INFANT FEEDING PRACTICES AND
SOCIAL STRUCTURES

Infant feeding practices have been found to vary with the mothers' social structures (White et al., 1992; Foster et al., 1997; Nadesan & Sotirin, 1998; Guttman & Zimmerman, 2000; Li & Grummer-Strawn, 2002; Bailey et al., 2004; Cricco-Lizza, 2004, 2005). Mothers' socio-demographic characteristics which are positively associated with higher breastfeeding rates include non-white ethnicity (Jacobson et al., 1991; Robinson et al., 1993; Timbo et al., 1996; Wiemann et al., 1998; Li & Grummer-Strawn, 2002; Beal et al., 2003; Cricco-Lizza, 2005), higher educational status (Quarles et al., 1994; Giugliani et al., 1994; Spisak & Gross, 1991; Scott & Binns, 1999), older maternal age (Gabriel et al., 1986; Jacobson et al., 1991; Giugliani et al., 1994), and being married (Giugliani et al., 1994; Institute of Medicine, 1991). The recent review of the incidence and duration of breastfeeding for full-term infants in Canada, United States, Europe, and Australia (Callen & Pinelli, 2004: 285) shows that "women who initiate and continue to breastfeed are older, married, better educated, and have higher family incomes than women who do not breastfeed."

Breastfeeding rates among low-income mothers tend to be lower than those of the middle-class, higher income mothers (Eckhardt & Hendershot, 1984; Gabriel et al., 1986; Ryan & Martinez, 1989; Kistin et al., 1990; Buxton et al., 1991; Ryan et al., 1991; Brent et al., 1995; Ross Laboratories, 1995; Guttman & Zimmerman, 2000; Bailey et al., 2004; Cricco-Lizza, 2004, 2005). Although breastfeeding has been extensively promoted, breastfeeding rates among socio-economically disadvantaged mothers continue to be about 35 percentage points below the recommended levels (Grossman et al., 1989; Cunningham et al., 1991; Jacobson et al., 1991; Walker, 1993; National Center for Health Statistics, 1996; Guttman & Zimmerman, 2000; Li & Grummer-Strawn, 2002; Bailey et al., 2004; Cricco-Lizza, 2004, 2005).

Nurit Guttman and Deena Zimmerman (2000: 1468) reveal in their study that breastfeeding, for low-income mothers, has "the connotation of social class deprivation." Breastfeeding was regarded "as a luxury, an inconvenience, and as distasteful" among the working-class mothers in their study of breastfeeding choices among women in different income categories (Guttman & Zimmerman, 2000). One working-class woman portrayed a breastfeeding mother as someone who "has a lot of time on her hands." The comment of the working-class mother represented "a social distinction that allocates the material luxuries of breastfeeding to middle class mothers." Many low-income women contended that women, who were in a more privileged position than themselves, would find it easier to breastfeed. Thus, for the working-class women, the notion that breastfeeding is good for the baby and that good mothers should breastfeed may result in "tensions" more than pleasure. As Guttman and Zimmerman (2000: 1457) contend, feeding young infants today presents women with not only choices and desires, but also obligations and constraints. Ironically, the working-class women who wished to breastfeed received little social support from their family and friends. This was due to a shared perception that breastfeeding was inappropriate, or even "nasty."

As Majia Nadesan and Patty Sotirin (1998: 223–4) argue, the tensions organized around breast- and bottle-feeding underlines "the material and social distinctions under patriarchal, capitalist orders." They suggest that material and class structures influence women's decisions to breast- or bottle-feed. As Nadesan and Sotirin (1998: 223–4) point out, the middle-class women have a choice to stay at home with her children or to work. They are able to take longer maternity leaves or choose to work on a flexible schedule. Those who work may have better access to a private space for breast-pumping. Clearly, these women are more likely to breastfeed. On the contrary and all too often, the employments of the working-class women are concentrated in "gender-stratified fields" which have "less worker autonomy, less break time, and less economic flexibility." These women would then be more likely not to initiate or continue breastfeeding. As such, Nadesan and Sotirin (1998: 223–4) argue, breastfeeding "performs class as well as gender."

I contend that breastfeeding not only performs class and gender, but also ethnicity (see Timbo et al., 1996; Wiemann et al., 1998; Li & Grummer-Strawn, 2002; Beal et al., 2003; Cricco-Lizza, 2004, 2005). Ruowei Li and Laurence Grummer-Strawn (2002), who examined breastfeeding rates among women from different socio-economic and racial backgrounds in the United States, found that 60 percent of the breastfed children were from non-Hispanic white mothers whereas only 26 percent of black children had been breastfed. Black infants also had a lower rate of exclusive breastfeeding at 4 months than white infants. In their study, they conclude that black mothers had consistently lower breastfeeding rates than white mothers regardless of their socio-demographic levels. In addition, significant differences between high and low socio-economic classes among black women clearly indicates that social class status has a major influence on breastfeeding practices among black mothers. Roberta Cricco-Lizza (2004, 2005: 526), in her study with black women attending a WIC (BWEW) clinic in New York,[1] found that bottle-feeding was commonly practiced by these women. Infant feeding beliefs of these women were a reflection of their lived experiences: "a preponderance of loss and daily stress in their everyday lives" and their "experiences with financial hardship, abuse, discrimination, and fears of safety throughout pregnancy and the postpartum." These women also received little education and support from health professionals during their pregnancy and postpartum care. It is not surprising then to see low rates of breastfeeding among these women.

In Thailand, this situation is reversed. It has been a consistent pattern in Thailand that rural poor women tend to initiate and prolong breastfeeding in comparison to urban and educated Thai women (Knodel et al., 1990; Yimyam, 1997). In John Knodel and others' work, they found that urban women breastfed their children for a shorter period than rural mothers and only a small number of rural women did not breastfeed their infants. Knodel and colleagues (1990) also found regional differentials in breastfeeding patterns. The shortest duration of breastfeeding was found among children in Bangkok, the capital and most modern city in Thailand. Knodel and colleagues (1990: 148) conclude in their study that there are several social and economic influences that have discouraged breastfeeding practices among urban educated women. These include "the rising level of education of women in the reproductive age groups, urbanization and increasing labour force activity among women outside of agriculture."

The results of John Knodel and others (1990) are in line with those of Somchai Durongdej (1991), who conducted a large-scale study on infant feeding patterns in Bangkok. Durongdej (1991: 12) found that "older mothers and mothers born in Bangkok are less likely to initiate breastfeeding. Bangkok born mothers are also likely to stop breastfeeding earlier as are mothers from higher income families and mothers of lower parity . . . The medium duration of breastfeeding from the sample is just over six months." Interestingly, Durongdej (1991) also found that women who had a paid employment often had higher educational and income levels. Hence, they were more able to obtain suitable supplementary foods for their infants.

The situation in Thailand is also similar to that in Indonesia. In Valerie Hull and others' study (1990: 627) in Indonesia, they found that past durations of breastfeeding declined with education, and breastfeeding durations were shorter among employed women.

> Breast-feeding is not, however, always in step with the forces of modernization. In many contemporary developing countries, breast-feeding is typically shorter for more educated, affluent and younger women. (Hull et al., 1990: 625)

The highly educated women believed that breastfeeding might ruin the shape of their breasts. They were also concerned that they might have insufficient breast milk. Hull and colleagues (1990) also found that only a small number of women were not breastfeeding because they had to go back to work. The common reasons tended to concentrate on problems associated with breastfeeding such as nipple soreness, engorged or sore breasts, and a perception of insufficient breast milk. In some cases, women did not initiate breastfeeding because their infants were premature or weak, or because the mother did not feel well. Interestingly, Hull and others (1990: 632) conclude their study that "the women who were not breast-feeding were predominantly the victims of inadequate knowledge and poor breast-feeding management rather than women who made a voluntary choice based on sound advice."

In this chapter, I shall also show that rural poor women in Northern Thailand initiate and continue breastfeeding longer than those in an urban setting of Chiang Mai City.

EMPLOYMENT AND BREASTFEEDING PRACTICES

Maternal employment outside the home is an important factor in the decline of breastfeeding in many countries in the past several decades (Wright et al., 1993; Van Esterik & Menon, 1996; Blum, 1999; Yimyam et al., 1999; Galtry, 2003; Yimyam & Morrow, 2003; Dykes, 2005). Fiona Dykes (2005: 2291) points out that globally, increasing numbers of women will return to paid employment during early motherhood. This common pattern, Dykes (2005: 2291) argues, "creates many dilemmas for women as they juggle the demands upon their time and bodies" (see also Blum, 1999, Yimyam et al., 1999; Galtry, 2003; Yimyam & Morrow, 2003). Working is seen as being incompatible with breastfeeding among mothers and their families in many societies (Durongdej, 1991; Yimyam, 1997; Yimyam et al., 1999; Guttman & Zimmerman, 2000; Yimyam & Morrow, 2003). Susanha Yimyam and colleagues (1999: 9571) contend, "breastfeeding becomes increasingly complex when women are employed, especially outside the home." It has been found that women who either choose to work, or for many poor women who must return to work for financial survival, tend to have a shorter period of feeding than those who do not work (Richter et al., 1992; Hills-Bonczyk et al., 1993; Yimyam, 1997; Guttman & Zimmerman, 2000; Yimyam & Morrow, 2003).

Susanha Yimyam and Martha Morrow (1999), for example, point out in their work with Thai women in Northern Thailand that returning to paid employment negatively influenced the rate and duration of breastfeeding. They report that "at 6 months postpartum, women who worked inside the home breastfed more than those working in the formal sector at jobs with inflexible hours (home, 80%; public sector, 37%; private sector, 39%)." Women who had to work outside the home for a long period and those who had shift jobs faced many challenges and problems to continue breastfeeding. Most abandoned it within one month of returning to paid work. In his study in Bangkok, Thailand, Somchai Durongdej (1991: 14) too found that work outside the home was an important influence on infant feeding practices for the subgroup of women who are so employed. The overall effect was the increased introduction of early bottle-feeding and the decrease of breastfeeding duration.

Patricia Romito and Marie-Joséphe Saurel-Cubizolles (1996), in their study in a small town in Italy, have also suggested another interesting pattern of breastfeeding and employment. They found the effect of the length of maternity leave on breastfeeding duration; the longer the leave, the longer mothers breastfed their infants. One third of mothers continued to breastfeed their infants after the resumption of their employment. This confirms that many working mothers had high motivation to continue breastfeeding. Of those who stayed at home longer, many suggested that they would be happy to go back to work but still continue to breastfeed their babies in the morning and in the afternoon. Romito and Saurel-Cubizolles (1996) suggest that their findings were positive and this was due to the social context of Italy, particularly a generous maternity leave provided for new mothers. This is also what Philipona (1994) has shown in her study in Norway, where the number of employed mothers is high. Many women in her study had important political positions, and the incidence and duration of breastfeeding was the highest in the developed world (see also Liesto et al., 1988; Rasmussen & Moss, 1993). This is because, as Philipona (1994) contends, maternity leave is generous in this society.

Literature in Western societies suggests that women who are employed in high status jobs as professionals tend to combine more working with breastfeeding than women who are not working (Kurinu et al., 1989; Hills-Bonczyk et al., 1993). Natalie Kurinu and others (1989) found that women in professional employment had a longer period of breastfeeding than women in non-professional positions such as those in the sales or technical (Yimyam, 1997: 32). This is because, Yimyam (1997: 32) argues, "women working as professionals have greater flexibility and more control over their work environment." And, this allows them to have "a more satisfactory relationship between the demands of employment and infant feeding" (cf. Kurinu et al., 1989; Morse et al., 1989; Hills-Bonczyk et al., 1993).

The woman's ability to combine employment and breastfeeding, Jan Morse and colleagues (1989) suggest, is dependent on the nature of their employment or work. Rural work in, for example, agricultural or marketing industries seems to be compatible with breastfeeding and child care in general. Most mothers can keep their infants while working (Selvaratnam, 1988; Podhisita et al., 1990). But, for women working in the formal and urban settings, breastfeeding becomes problematic, as their work occurs outside the home, and it is more difficult to balance the demands placed on them. This seems to be more marked within the formal sector where child-care provision is not available.

Susanha Yimyam (1997: 247, original emphasis) also clearly documents in her research on breastfeeding patterns in northern Thailand, that her study "present[s] a compelling argument that it is not **employment** per se, but **inflexible hours of work** and **separation from the infant** which make the crucial difference to breastfeeding among employed women." This is in line with the argument of Penny van Esterik and Ted Greiner (1981) who suggest that employment may not be an important factor, but that the conditions in the work environment impact breastfeeding among Thai women.

Despite general evidence suggesting that paid employment had negative impacts on the duration of breastfeeding, some studies have interestingly revealed that maternal employment is associated with a longer period of breastfeeding (Kurinu et al., 1989; O'Gara, 1989; Wright et al., 1993; Ross Laboratories, 1995). Employed women practised mixed-feeding for longer periods of time. Anne Wright and others (1993) found in their study with Navajo women that mothers who started work outside the home after three months initiated formula feeding later and breastfed longer than others, including unemployed mothers. They suggest that paid employment may not influence duration if breastfeeding is firmly established before mothers return to work. Furthermore, women who work outside the home may have higher motivation to continue breastfeeding for a longer period, as breastfeeding permits the maintenance of intimacy with their infants after separation during the day (Wright et al., 1993: 275). Wright and colleagues (1993) suggest that breastfeeding rates among employed Navajo women equal or exceed those of other women when employment is postponed despite the fact that working is seen as a barrier to breastfeeding. As such, maternal employment may influence breastfeeding only under some circumstances.

BREAST- AND BOTTLE-FEEDING: MORAL AND DEVIANT MOTHERS

The dominant idea that "breast is best" (Stanway & Stanway, 1978) is pervasive in literature on infant feeding patterns and in policy and health promotion attempting to educate women about their infant feeding practices (Nadesan & Sotirin, 1998; Murphy, 1999; Guttman & Zimmerman, 2000; Sheehan, 2006). Within the lay population, this idea is also promulgated. Due to the societal perception of the superiority of breastfeeding, as Elizabeth Murphy (1999: 187) contends, mothers' intention not to breastfeed their babies may tarnish the "moral status" of motherhood. By choosing to bottle-feed their infants, a mother is subjected to the accusation that she is a "bad" mother, who "places her own needs, preferences or conveniences above her baby's welfare" (Murphy, 1999: 187). On the contrary, the "good mother" is "deemed to be one who prioritises her child's needs, even (or perhaps especially) where this entails personal inconvenience or distress" (Murphy, 1999: 187-188), such as trying to breastfeed against many obstacles.

Motherhood, Majia Nadesan and Patty Sotirin (1998: 221) contend, is "often represented as the ultimate expression of womanhood while breast-feeding is represented as the ultimate experience of motherhood." Because of this, as Elizabeth Murphy (1999: 188) suggests, the decision to bottle-feed is likely to be considered as "questionable" (McHugh, 1970).

> It leaves women open to the charge of being a poor mother, in short, of maternal deviance. The intention to formula feed threatens women's claims to qualities such as selflessness, wisdom, responsibility and far-sightedness all of which are widely seen as evidence of being a 'good mother' (Murphy, 1999: 188).

Nurit Guttman and Deena Zimmerman (2000: 1458) argue that "the discourses on motherhood, nurture, naturalness and modernity" has created the moral image of breastfeeding. As Sarah Earle (2000: 327) points out in her study with women in Coventry, England, women perceived breastfeeding as natural. A woman who did not breastfeed was perceived as "a horrible mother." As such, women who intend to bottle-feed their infants open themselves to a charge of deviance (Goffman, 1963) or "immoral mothers" (Liamputtong, 2006).

Deviance, according to Murphy (1999: 189), "involves a charge that public morality is being violated" and in the case of infant feeding, mothers break the rules of infant feeding. But more than that, as Murphy (1999: 188) theorises, "the moral mother is not simply one who follows the rules. Rather, she is one who follows the rules *knowingly.*" Hence, simply breaking the rules does not make the mother deviant, but "her deviance rests upon a judgement that she has broken the rules *knowingly*" (McHugh, 1970: 188, original emphasis). In the case of infant feeding, mothers who choose not to breastfeed their infants and know very well about the likely impacts of the practice on infant's health are potentially subject to the charge of deviance as "immoral mothers."

Social rules, Gresham Sykes and David Matza (1957: 666, original emphasis) argue, are "*qualified* guides to action." The charge of being immoral or deviant mothers, Murphy contends "is always defeasible in the sense that it is open to the possibility of refutation." Robert Dingwall (1976) suggests this possibility is dependent on the ability of the individual to appeal to some "possible grounds for refuting the accusation." Therefore, Elizabeth Murphy (1999: 189–190) suggests, despite the fact that breastfeeding is socially constructed as "the optimal method of infant feeding" which has ramifications for the judgement of moral motherhood, "the rule that 'good mothers breast-feed' is not so rigid as to be binding under all circumstance." There appears to be some possibilities for women who intend to bottle-feed to "challenge or resist the interpretation of their behaviour as morally sanctionable." To do so, Sykes and Matza (1957) and Marvin Scott and Standford Lyman (1963) suggest the use of "techniques of neutralisation," particularly "justification." According to Scott and Lyman (1963) and Murphy (1999: 190), justification involves "an acceptance that the act is deviant, while seeking to rebut any suggestion that it is therefore morally or socially sanctionable."

In relation to infant feeding, however, Murphy (1999: 190) contends, women who intend to bottle-feed must prove that, while it breaks the rule, it is nonetheless justified. When the decision to formula feed her baby is questioned, a mother must justify that her intention is "non-conventional"; that is "she could not have done otherwise." She has no other choices and hence her intention should not be sanctioned since it can be justified. Therefore, the charge of deviance should be abolished. As Anne Wright and colleagues (1993: 262) contend, when breastfeeding is socially valued in societies, women choosing not to breastfeed may use socially and culturally acceptable grounds for their actions, such as the need to work in a paid employment and having insufficient milk to justify their actions. This will help them to escape being seen as "bad mothers."

In this chapter, I shall show that the morality of breastfeeding is also pervasive among Thai women in Northern Thailand. I shall also examine the ways in which women talk about their accounts/stories which are used to deny the charge that their choices are deemed deviant, even though they might bottle-feed their infants.

"BREAST IS BEST" NOTION: WOMEN'S ACCOUNTS

There is no doubt that the women in my study perceived breast milk as the best food for their newborn and young infants (cf. Van Esterik, 1988; Vong-Ek, 1993; Family Health Division, 1994; Yimyam, 1997; Liamputtong Rice & Naksook, 2001). It is said that breast milk contains antibiotics and all nutrients that could not be equalled by consuming all the five food groups. Women remarked that only breast milk contains all the goodness that newborn and young infants need. Pimpilai, an urban educated woman, provided the following explanation when asked about breast milk:

> Mother's milk is best as it provides good immunity to the baby, so that the baby will have a high resistance to ill health and diseases. People say that breastfed

babies will have a good resistance and immunity and these children will not get sick or catch a cold easily.

Saijai, an urban middle-class woman, similarly remarked:

> I have been breastfeeding for 10 months. I have read many books and they all say that breast milk is best for the baby. I wanted my baby to get all the best things in her life and so I breastfeed her.

Not only breast milk provides the best sort of nutrients to an infant, the act of breastfeeding also provides warmth and psychological well-being to their newborn as well. Wilai, an urban educated woman, had some interesting remarks about breastfeeding. She suggested that the nutrients in infant formula nowadays is more or less similar to breast milk, but the act of breastfeeding in fact provides more closeness, warmth, and emotional well-being to both the mother and her newborn. Similarly, Sumalee, a rural woman, reflected on her belief about breast milk that:

> I think the best food for my baby is mother's milk. It is the purest form of food that screens from our own body. The baby will receive warmth and love from a mother. Mother's goodness will then be passed onto the baby through breast milk. And, this is the best way for the baby to be passed on good stuff from us as mothers.

When prompted about bottle-feeding, Sumalee remarked that:

> With bottle-feeding, even though we feed the baby ourself, it is not the same as feeding the baby from our body. It is like putting cow's milk into the baby's body. When we breastfeed, we can cuddle the baby, we can hold the baby close to our body. But, it is not the same when we use the bottle. We might cuddle the baby, but it does not give me the same sort of feelings like breastfeeding. So, feeding the baby by a bottle is not the same as feeding from our breasts because it is not coming out from our own bodies.

Of interest is the perception among rural or poor women who contended that breast milk not only makes the infant strong and healthy, it was also financially sound. Mothers did not have to spend money on buying infant formula. This is clearly seen in the account given by Isara, a rural poor woman who breastfed her infant for three months. The infant became very ill and had to be hospitalized. While in hospital, the nursing staff bottle-fed him, and as a result her breast milk dried up. In Isara's mind, this was unfortunate for not only her infant, but also for her financial situation, as now she had to find money to purchase infant formula for her baby, rather than being able to save money for other necessities needed in the family. Kesara, another rural poor woman, suggested similarly, when she said:

> Mother's milk is the best milk for the baby. Mother can relax at home as she does not have to run around doing the bottles. If you use an infant formula, it is not economical. Nowadays, money is so hard to obtain, so feeding with breast milk is best.

Orachorn, also a rural poor woman, contended that breast milk was not only best for her babies, but because of her financial circumstances, she had no other option. She gave us this explanation:

> I breastfed my babies, all of them, because what else I could feed them apart from breast milk. I am not in a position to buy any infant food to give them. Breastfeeding was the only option I had.

The economic benefit of breastfeeding was also remarked by urban poor women. Wasana remarked about breast milk that:

> It is more beneficial than bottle milk. I feel that it provides more emotional connection between a mother and her baby. It allows an opportunity to have a close bodily contact with the baby. And, we don't have to spend money on buying the milk either.

Of note is the fact that more rural poor women initiated and continued breast-feeding for a long period of time. This was partly due to their financial constraints as well as their understanding of the goodness of breast milk.

Others talked about the hygienic aspect of breastfeeding. They would compare this with that of bottle-feeding.

> I believe breast milk is best because if we bottle-feed, we have to make up the bottles and they may not be clean enough and this will create the likelihood of the baby getting germs more than from mother's milk. This is why people say mother's milk is the best for her baby. (Sirin, an urban educated woman)

Women made sense of the benefit of breast milk from their lived experiences with breastfeeding and other feeding methods. Sinjai, an urban educated woman, compared the health of her two children; one was bottle-fed and another breastfed:

> As far as I can see is that a breastfed baby is much healthier and stronger than a formula-fed baby. [Nong Toy] is not that strong, when he was a little baby, he was very thin and always had some sort of ill health like it was very easy for him to get a cold or diarrhoea. He was formula fed. But [Nong Tu] who was breast-

fed is always healthy; never got sick. I can easily see the differences between them.

BREAST MILK: *LUAD NAI OK*—MOTHER'S BLOOD AND MOTHER/CHILD CONNECTION

Breastfeeding, Penny van Esterik (1988, 1989) suggests, is perceived as "a holistic and integrated activity" within a more traditional society like Thailand. Indeed, as Fiona Dykes (2005: 2287) points out, within traditional communities, breastfeeding is illustrated "as entirely relationally orientated with absence of any dichotomy between the baby's nutritional and emotional needs." The women in Dykes's study (2005: 2286) made reference to "intimacy, closeness and nurture, seeing breastfeeding as much more than providing breast milk to the baby." Sushila Zeitlyn and Rabeya Rowshan (1997) theorise that through breastfeeding, women and their breastfed children are "interconnected and indivisible." This is clearly reflected in the Thai women's discourses regarding the origin of breast milk. The notion that breast milk is best stems largely from a traditional belief among Thai people that it is produced from the blood of the mother. Often, breast milk is referred to as *luad nai ok*, literally meaning "blood from mother's chest." It symbolises sacrifice and maternal love of a mother toward her infant.

> Breast milk comes from the blood of a mother; it is *luad nai ok*, *luad* [blood] which is produced in her *ok* [chest]. (Saijai, an urban middle-class woman)

Zeitlyn and Rowshan (1997) point out that, Bangladeshi women see the connection between a mother and a child through breastfeeding. In a similar manner, Sumalee, a rural woman, contended that:

> Breast milk comes from our own blood; it is filtered from our blood—mother's blood. This is why there is always a strong connection between a mother and her child.

Suriya, a rural poor woman, remarked that:

> The best milk for a baby is mother's milk. It is much better than anything else because it provides warmth and closeness to the baby, much more than bottle-feeding, because mother's milk is made from the mother's blood.

The interconnectedness between mothers and infants can be seen from an interesting account given by Saijai, an urban middle-class woman. In this case, it deserves our attention. Saijai has been breastfeeding her baby for ten months. When she had to return to work, she twice tried to wean the baby from breastfeeding. Both attempts failed, according to her. She elaborated on these attempts:

> I tried to wean him twice. When he was about seven months old, I stopped him from my breast, but he would cry until he vomited. Once he cried to the point that he was in shock. It was like his cry was frozen. I was so sorry for the baby and said to myself I would not wean him. So, I continued breastfeeding. You should see his face when I put him back on my breast. Even it was just a short suck, he was smiling and I was feeling so sorry for him. I was in tears. How could I, as a mother, wean my baby when he is like this?

My interpretation is that breastfed mothers, as Elizabeth Murphy (1999: 200) suggests, "simultaneously display adequate maternal knowledge (that 'breast is best') and appropriate maternal morality (that they would prioritise the baby's welfare)." Women knew very well what was best for their babies, and they intended to do so. As such, as Murphy (1999: 201) suggests, "breast-feeding was treated not only compatible with, but indeed, indicative of, maternal morality."

Some women would suggest that breast milk is made from food a mother consumes during the *yu duan* (confinement) period (see chapter 5). The consumed food is made into the mother's blood and then turned into breast milk (cf. Zeitlyn & Rowshan, 1997; Liamputtong & Naksook, 2001). Hence, women would be particularly cautious about food consumption during the first month after birth, as it could affect the health of their infants. Clearly, this is a reflection of the mother-baby connection through breastfeeding. Isara, a rural poor woman, told us that:

> Breast milk is from our own blood; our blood is filtered and made into breast milk. So, whatever we eat during lactation will get into the baby's body too; like if we eat hot food, the baby might have a stomach ache. So, we have to be careful with what we eat during the first month. I would *kam kin*—restrict myself with diet during this time; things like hot food or pickles I would not eat during *yu duan* at all.

Malai, a rural woman, similarly remarked on this that:

> Breast milk is made from our blood; the blood is filtered into milk for the baby. If we eat good food during confinement, it will get into the breast milk. So, it is like our baby will receive the best possible food from our body.

But, for some well-off women, the consumption of good food must start early. Sinjai volunteered that:

Breast milk is from the food we eat. We have to nourish our bodies; make our bodies healthy and strong. It will help us to produce good blood and then this blood will turn into breast milk for the baby. This is why we have to make sure that we eat good food from when we become pregnant.

On the contrary, many poor women would feel that due to their poverty, their food intake was not sufficient and nutritious enough for them to produce good breast milk for their babies. As such, their babies might not receive good milk, and hence, this might affect their connection with their babies.

The mother [she] did not have good food to eat during pregnancy; only rice and sweet potatoes. How could the baby get good breast milk then? When I was pregnant, I only had rice noodle curry [cheap dish to prepare], so my baby did not get good nutritious food either. I was not in good health, and so the baby would not be born healthy. I did not have the chance to drink milk or any other nutritious food and this is because I am poor. I live in poverty, hence I could not live and eat well and this affected the quality of breast milk. (Malai, a rural poor woman)

MOTHERS' DECISION TO BOTTLE-FEED

Despite their knowledge about the goodness of breast milk, several mothers in my study decided to bottle-feed their infants. Araya, an urban educated woman, when asked what she believed to be the best food for a new born infant, expressed her idea that: "Of course, mother's milk because breast milk is beneficial as mothers will eat all the good things in order to produce breast milk for our babies." But, when asked if she breastfed her newborn, she said "No, my baby is having a bottle." Her main reason was:

I did not have enough milk. At first, I did have some as I stimulated my breasts but because I had a problem with my cut from my caesarean birth, I could not feed the baby. I then started feeding him with infant formula.

For some women, a mixed feeding method was adopted for practical reasons such as the need to leave the baby with others due to commitments that they needed to attend to as part of their living reality. Pimpan, a rural woman, told us that she has breastfed the second baby for eleven months now, but she also gave the baby infant formula as a supplement. She had to attend to many tasks and if she only breastfed the baby, the baby would be clingy and it would not be practical for her to do her work properly. If the baby was accustomed to taking infant formula as well, she could leave the baby with a family member while she was doing something else.

There were two major reasons that the women in this study used to justify their decisions to bottle-feed their infants.

THE "NOT ENOUGH MILK" SYNDROME

Breastfeeding is full of contradictions. As Sushila Zeitlyn and Robeya Rowshan (1997: 57) point out, despite the fact that breast milk is important for child survival, "insufficient milk" is a commonly reported phenomenon, particularly among urban middle-class and educated women in many parts of the world (see Tully & Dewey, 1985; Hill, 1991; Hillervik-Lindquist, 1991; Marchand & Morrow, 1994; World Health Organization, 1996; Beasley et al., 1998; Dykes & Williams, 1999; Murphy, 2000; Abel et al., 2001; Dykes, 2002, 2005; Hamlyn et al., 2002; Moffat, 2002). Often, insufficient milk is used as a justification for many women to progress to bottle-feeding (Murphy, 2000; Dykes, 2005).

In Fiona Dykes's study (2005: 2287) the most striking and consistent theme that she found was that women lacked confidence and trust in their bodies. Women did not feel confident in their abilities to produce enough milk or the right quality milk. This lack of confidence was expressed not only by the women themselves, but was also obvious amongst the midwives. This is in a similar vein to the findings of Zeitlyn and Rowshan (1997: 58), in their research on insufficient milk in Bangladesh, who found that "breastmilk is regarded with ambivalence." Both mothers and health professionals often gave "insufficient milk" as a reason for not breastfeeding.

As Zeitlyn and Rowshan (1997: 63) point out in their study, women believed that their babies did not have enough breast milk and often the women would remark that "their milk 'dried up' or that the baby cried and was believed to be hungry." Some women remarked that breast milk did not "'satisfy' their infants or 'fill' their stomachs." That unsettled behaviors of their infants were associated with the women's perceptions of insufficient milk are also evident in other studies (see Hillervick-Linquist, 1991; Beasley et al., 1998; Dykes & Williams, 1999; Hamlyn et al., 2002; Moffat, 2002; Dykes, 2005). Susanha Yimyam (1997) also suggests that the most common breastfeeding problems given by Thai women in her study was due to insufficient milk. In my study, despite women's intention to breastfeed and for most, they attempted to do so for a long period of time, in reality, many could not do this. Sumalee, a rural woman, provided a clear account about the goodness of breastfeeding (see earlier section), but she was only able to breastfeed for two months, and it was not exclusive either. She adopted a mixed method. She defended herself as not only due to having "insufficient milk," but also the physiology of her nipples and the consequences of taking contraceptive pills.

I managed to breastfeed my baby for 2 months because I used a mixed method. The baby was always hungry; I could tell because she always curled her lips and sucked the air, and this indicated that she was hungry. I did not have enough milk to feed her; it did not really come out even she was sucking. My nipples were very short too, so it was hard for her to grasp. When she could not suck, she would cry and I felt sorry for her. So, I gave her some formula after breast-feeding. By the end of the second month, my milk was totally dried up. I think it was also because I was taking the Pill as well.

All too often, as Dykes (2005: 2287) points out, women's bodies have been seen as "weak, defective and deeply untrustworthy" and hence "denigrated." This has led women to think that their bodies are not suited to breastfeeding (see also Martin, 1992; Davis-Floyd, 1992, 1994; Blum, 1993; Duden, 1993; Shildrick, 1997; Dykes, 2002, 2005). Due to this, breastfeeding may be seen "as something which will be difficult (or impossible) to achieve successfully" (Earle, 2000: 326) by women. Panee Vong-Ek (1993) and Fiona Dykes (2002, 2005) argue that beliefs in insufficient milk may lead women to adopt formula feeding or weaning of breast milk. This has been demonstrated by some of the women in this study.

Paid Work and Breastfeeding

Maternity leave entitlement in Thailand is not very generous, nor uniform across the work forces (cf. Romito and Saurel-Cubizolles, 1996 for maternity leave legislation in Italy). As Susanha Yimyam and others (1999: 958) contend, "there is no comprehensive, universal legislation protecting the breastfeeding rights of employed women and few private companies or government agencies provide regular support in this sphere." It has been observed that only women who work in the government sector or some privileged business sectors may receive a better deal of maternity leave than those working in the private sector or factories. The current legislation regarding maternity leave in Thailand was enacted in May 1993 (Yimyam, 1997; Yimyam & Morrow, 2003). For those who are Thai government and state enterprises employees, they are entitled to ninety days maternity leave with full pay. However, women may request a further 180 days unpaid personal leave for childrearing. For those in the private sector, if they are permanent employees, they will be given ninety days maternity leave with pay. According to the Labour Protection Law, employers are to be paid up to forty-five days from their own funds and the other forty-five days can be claimed from the national Social Security Fund, to which the employees have also contributed (Yimyam, 1997). For many women, who work as casual, part-time, and subcontract workers, or those who work on a daily basis and for small businesses, do not have access to maternity leave at all (Van Esterik, 1988; Richter et al., 1992; Yinyam, 1997; Yimyam & Morrow, 2003). As such, it is clear that the ability of mothers to breastfeed their babies is dependent upon "regulations on maternity leave time." In a study that examined the impact of the duration of postnatal leave and other factors on the pattern of breastfeeding amongst 790 public employees in Bangkok (Boonwanich, 1993), it was found that about 50 percent of the babies were weaned by the completion of maternity leave of the mothers. Those who took leave of less than ninety days, weaned their babies at the period between one and two months. These mothers, as Boonwanich suggested, initiated early weaning as a way to prepare their babies to take infant formula from a child-care provider. In Yimyam and colleagues' work (1999), they discovered that most women in their study clearly wanted to combine work and breastfeeding. However, many found the demands of these simultaneous roles problematic. Because of the need to combine work and breastfeeding, many mothers weaned their children prematurely.

Returning to work, Susanha Yimyam (1997: 50) contends, is given by many women as their reason for weaning, including Northern Thai mothers (see also Winikoff et al., 1988; Jackson et al., 1992; Richter et al., 1992; Yimyam & Morrow, 2003; Dykes, 2005). In my study, women who returned to work early could not continue their breastfeeding. This was problematic for some poor women who needed to return to work soon after their maternity leave entitlement ceased. Naree, an urban poor woman, had to leave her youngest infant with her oldest daughter who was to feed the baby with infant formula. The baby refused the bottle and did not thrive. Naree remarked:

> I had to go to work, but the baby would refuse the bottle. I tried infant formula but he would not take it. We had to leave him to cry and he cried until he eventually had to start taking the bottle. So, he was so thin, even now he is still thin. This is the problem for me with feeding because I had to return to work.

But, this was also problematic for some urban women. Manee breastfed her first child for only one month, but could do so for three months with her second child. Both short periods of breastfeeding were results of her limited maternity leave. She remarked:

> My first baby was breastfed for only one month, as that was all the leave I could get. My second baby was able to take breast milk for three months as I was able to take three months leave. After that they both had to take the bottle.

Due to financial needs, women returned to work, and hence these women made their decisions to bottle-feed. Women's decisions to bottle-feed, Murphy (1999: 194) suggests, is a clear indication of their justification that they are indeed good mothers; mothers who would do anything to ensure "a reliable supply of food" for their infants. This is further evidenced by the way the women managed their two roles. They attempted to do the best for their infants, as Manee told us:

> But, I tried to breastfeed them at night, so that I could continue breastfeeding until they were six or seven months old.

For some mothers, however, returning to work might not extensively interfere with their breastfeeding. It seems, as Yimyam (1997: 33) points out, the type and location of work and the opportunity for mothers to make contact with infants during working hours determined infant feeding behavior amongst mothers in my study. Clearly, mothers' access to their infants during working hours assisted them to continue breastfeeding (Winikoff & Castle, 1988; WHO, 1993; Yimyam & Morrow, 2003). Wilai, an urban educated woman, was able to continue breastfeeding for six months. The baby was placed in a child-care center belonged to her work place. She would go to feed the baby three times a day during her working hours. Wilai was fortunate in the sense that she was working at a place where child care was provided for staff and it was in a close proximity. But, even in Wilai's case, she had to gradually introduce the bottle to her child and by six months the child was ready to abandon breast milk. Wilai remarked:

> With my second baby, I continued to breastfeed her until 6 months. Even when she attended a child care, I continued to feed her. But, after three months of doing this, I started to give her infant formula. By 6 months, she did not want my breasts anymore; may be the milk did not flow as well as the bottle milk. So, she refused to take my breasts and that was the end of my breastfeeding career.

Warunee and Patanee, who both are urban educated women, continued to breastfeed their babies long after they returned to work. Similar to Wilai, they were able to access the child care organized within their work places, and this enabled them to breastfeed their babies during working hours.

Others would find their own practical solutions to enable them to combine breastfeeding and work. Most often, women use a mixed method of feeding; they would breastfeed their infants at night, while during the day, the infant was given a bottle at a child-care center, or if at home, by family members like a grandmother. Siriporn, an urban educated woman, returned to her work when both of her babies were three months old. In the first three months, she adopted an exclusive breastfeeding regime. She continued to breastfeed them at night for nine months with the first child and more than ten months for the second. At the time of our interview, she was still breastfeeding her second

baby. It seems that some women would continue to do what they could despite the need to resume work.

NOT BREASTFEEDING?
JUSTIFICATION OF MATERNAL MORALITY

As Elizabeth Murphy (2000: 309) contends, bottle-feeding is "presented as
compatible with the morality of motherhood," women who intended to bottle-
feed their babies in my study knew very well that their intention would be
likely to be seen as being "bad mothers." Their narratives, however, indicated
the trend to defend themselves that bottle-feeding is "wrong, bad, or irre-
sponsible." As such, by implication, they are not "bad mothers" (Murphy,
1999: 193). Bottle-feeding was used as an "accountable decision" (Scott &
Lyman, 1963) by the women in my study.

Murphy (1999: 194), in her study, found that women who decided to bottle-
feed attempted to show that "they cared too much to expose their babies to any
risk that food would not be available when required." These women claimed
that mothers who formula feed their babies should be seen as "good mothers."
By contrast, those who breastfeed "risk a culpable maternal behavior," as they
made their babies go hungry while they could prevent this by giving them formula substance. Good mothers, according to the women in Murphy's study,
should "ensure that their babies had a dependable, scientifically formulated
source of food." To these women, a good mother can achieve in a different
way (Murphy, 1999: 197).

Likewise, the women in my study who bottle-fed or adopted a mixed method
of feeding would defend themselves that they did so because of their love and
concern about the health and well-being of their babies. If they were unable to
produce enough breast milk, and if they did not initiate bottle-feeding, the infant might not survive or thrive well. With the formula, many women perceived
that it contained similar good nutrients to breast milk. It was better to have milk
to feed their babies, whatever the milk might be. These women would see that
their intention to bottle-feed was beneficial to their infants, and this was the reflection of maternal love. Hence, they would still be seen as being good mothers despite bottle-feeding their infants. Prapaporn, an urban educated woman,
asserted that:

> I used a mixedfeeding pattern. I fed the baby with infant formula after breast
> milk because I did not have enough milk. The baby was frustrated and cried so
> I had to use the bottle to supplement breastfeeding. My nipples were small and
> this made it difficult for my baby to suck and I think this is why my milk did not
> really flow well. I could not leave the baby cry with hunger and hence I used

both milks. It is better this way if we can't produce enough milk for the baby
. . . If I had enough breast milk I would not give her the bottle.

As suggested above, many women in my study perceived that infant formula
contained similar good nutrients to breast milk. This is the way women justified their intentions and practices. As Murphy (1999: 196) points out in her
study too, that the women used this justification to challenge the fundamental belief that "breast is best." These women argued that "formula feeding was
not harmful." This is what Sykes and Matza (1957) and Scott and Lyman
(1963) define as "denials of injury." As one woman in Murphy's study (cited
in Murphy, 1999: 196) remarked, "there's the same nutrients in both . . . they
say breast milk is better because it's yours and it's nature . . . there's definitely
the same nutrients in both." To this mother, "the nutrient values of breast and
formula milk are identical and equally suitable for the baby," and this was in
contradiction to the opinion of health professionals.

This is not too surprising, however, if we consider the ads utilized by infant formula companies. As Rima Apple (1987: 42) points out, one ad by
Nestlé clearly articulated the benefit of infant formula:

> The Improved Nestlé's Milk Food, prepared with equal parts of fresh cow's
> milk and water, provides an ideal feeding for the normal infant-properly bal-
> anced in fat, protein, carbohydrate and mineral salt-and of excellent digestibil-
> ity. The carbohydrate—being a mixture of lactose, saccharose, maltose, dextrin
> and starch—modifies the milk ideally.

Women who adopted a mixed method would justify their practices and defend their good mother identity by insisting on giving breast milk to their infant prior to the bottle. This was the way to ensure that their infants would receive good food as much as possible. Darunee, an urban educated woman,
contended that:

> I would make sure that the baby took breast milk before the bottle. I would
> breastfeed until I felt that I would not have milk in my breasts then I would give
> the baby infant formula. The baby became used to bottle milk and would not
> want to take my breast, but I would insist on this. He did not like it, but I would
> persevere with it.

Pimpilai, an urban educated woman, justified her mixed method by saying
that:

> I believe that mother's milk is best, but if we can't produce enough milk for our
> babies, we then need to also give infant formula too. The baby should receive a
> well-balanced of quantity of milk. My milk was little; the baby only sucked a
> few times I would not have any more milk to feed him. No matter how hard I

tried to produce a lot of milk, I did not succeed. So, I felt sorry for my baby, as I could see that he was hungry.

DOCTOR KNOWS BEST:
ADVICE AND ENCOURAGEMENT FROM DOCTORS AND OTHER HEALTH PROFESSIONALS

The authoritative knowledge (Jordan, 1997), or privileged knowledge (Zeitlyn & Rowshan, 1997) of health professionals and particularly doctors abound in the accounts regarding infant feeding practices among the women in my study (see also Manderson, 1985; Millard, 1990; and chapter 2 in this volume). This is marked in relation to the promotion of "correct" or "proper" breastfeeding (see Lawrence, 1995; Dykes, 2005). In a more subtle way, as Sushila Zeitlyn and Rabeya Rowshan (1997: 58) contend, the "proper" breast-feeding promotion implicitly makes existing feeding patterns problematic, and hence requires "surveillance and correction by experts with privileged knowledge." Zeitlyn and Rowshan (1997: 56-57) also argue that despite the fact that breastfeeding is perceived as "a natural activity," it is also seen as one that could be improved on with the assistance of experts including doctors and other health professionals. In the Bangladeshi context, Zeitlyn and Rowshan (1997: 66) argue, "the legitimacy of professional experts is supported by claims of privileged knowledge about breast-feeding and the right of professionals to define what is 'natural' for infants and their mothers." In this section, I shall show that current discourses on breastfeeding provide health professionals with a venue for expressing changing ideas about motherhood in addition to confirming their authority.

It has been suggested that Thai mothers would discard colostrum, referred to as "yellow milk," due to a belief that colostrum is harmful to the newborn infant's health (Anuman Rajadhon, 1987; Winichagoon et al., 1992; Vong-Ek, 1993; Family Health Division, 1994; Yimyam, 1997; Liamputtong Rice & Naksook, 2001). This belief is also pervasive in many traditional societies (see Jellife & Jellife, 1978; Morse, 1984, 1985; Conton, 1985; Dettwyler, 1987; King & Ashworth, 1987; Fernandez & Popkin, 1988; Fishman et al., 1988; Morse et al., 1990; Gunnlaugsson & Einarsdottir, 1993; Liamputtong, 2002). But, this is contested in my study. Women, both rural poor and urban educated, believed strongly in the benefit of colostrum. It appears that this changed knowledge and perceptions of colostrum derived from the advice of doctors and other health professionals including nurses at hospitals or health care centres. Pimjai, a rural poor woman, when asked if her babies received colostrum, said:

When the babies were just born, they did get yellow milk [colostrum]. My doctor told me that it contains the best sort of food for the baby, as it has all sorts of vitamin in it, and so I should give it to the baby. So both of my babies did get the yellow milk; as soon as they were born, I put them on my breast.

When I asked Suriya, a rural woman, about her perception of colostrum, she remarked that colostrum is "the best of all food that a baby may take." This knowledge was passed on from the doctor at the hospital. Naree, an urban poor woman, told us that her youngest baby took colostrum from her breasts, and this was because her doctor recommended that it was not harmful to the baby. But, with her first child she did not give him colostrum.

I was afraid that my baby would have a stomach ache. Most people in my neighbourhood would discard colostrum because they said it was dirty milk and it would cause a stomach problem, so we have to squeeze it out. But, *samai ni* [nowadays], most doctors would tell us that we should feed the baby colostrum.

Women remarked that knowledge of breast milk and breastfeeding was passed on from health professionals. Women were educated in hospitals that breast milk would be best for their newborn infants. Ruchira, a rural woman, told us that health professionals at the hospital where she gave birth told her that breastfeeding would greatly benefit her baby, and for this reason she insisted on breastfeeding.

Not only was the knowledge of breastfeeding passed on by health professionals, but also the "right" or "proper" way of feeding their infants. Doctors always gave women advice regarding how to breastfeed their infants. Suriya, a rural poor woman, also remarked that when she was in hospital, the doctor told her to put her baby on her breasts soon after the baby was born. According to her doctor, this was to ensure that her baby would receive colostrum. Sinjai, an urban educated and financially secure woman, was unable to breastfeed her first baby. As the baby had a heart problem and was in an incubator in the first month of his life, he was unable to suck properly. He eventually was given a bottle. However, she managed to breastfeed her second baby for a year. She commenced breastfeeding soon after caesarean section and this was the advice given by her own doctor.

I fed [Nong Tu] for a long time; more than a year. As soon as I recovered in the recovery room, my doctor came to see me and he emphasised to me that I must breastfeed my baby. He was encouraging me to do so and he explained that the baby was still very little; she did not need a lot of milk, so I should not be worried that I would not have enough milk for her. At first I was worried because I could not see much milk from my breasts at all. But, what my doctor told me helped me not to worry and it was true, after I started breastfeed her, I had more milk. I would put her on my breasts often and did not give her any bottle at all. And, this is why I could continue breastfeeding for a long period of time.

Pimpilai, an urban educated woman, had difficulty with breastfeeding as she believed she did not have enough milk to feed the baby. But, by listening to the advice of her doctor, she was able to overcome this problem.

> My doctor told me to stimulate my breasts. He told me to put the baby on both breasts; ten minutes on the left and ten on the right, to swap over so that the baby could get breast milk from both breasts. He also said that if I did this, I would have equal size breasts. So, I followed his advice.

But, we also witnessed women who would resist the advice of health professionals. While in a minority, these women challenged the authority of professionals to define their good practices in infant feeding. Rather, the women argued that "mother knows best." Here, they adopted another kind of justification, theorized by Gresham Sykes and David Matza (1957: 668) as "condemning the condemners." Elizabeth Murphy (1999: 197) suggests, this requires the mothers to shift "the focus of attention from her own deviant acts to the motives and behaviours of those who disapprove." Warunee, an urban educated woman, believed strongly in the goodness of breast milk and insisted on exclusive breastfeeding. While she was still in hospital, a nurse recommended that she might consider giving the baby a bottle as well as breast milk, as it would be easier for her to manage her work and to wean the baby. The nurse adopted the "scientific motherhood" to "dissuade the woman from breastfeeding" (Nadesan & Sotirin, 1998: 224). But, she rejected this recommendation because her own circumstances would allow her to continue breastfeeding without any difficulty.

> I would not give her any bottle. The nurse suggested that I should give her both, taking turn between my milk and a formula. But, I refused that because I believed that my milk was the best for my baby. The nurse said I would have a problem weaning the baby if I insisted on breastfeeding. I did not think too much about it because I knew that I would put the baby at the child-care near work and I would manage with breastfeeding anyhow.

Feeding on schedule is a clear example of authoritative knowledge of health professionals. Feeding on schedule was recommended by health professionals in Thailand. Ann Millard (1990) asserts, women are educated to make distinctions between "on-demand feeding" and "by-the-clock" feeding. Millard (1990: 217) contends, "the clock has assumed a central location in breastfeeding advice." This is "a symbol of science, discipline, and the coordination of human effort." In her analysis of pediatric advice on breastfeeding, Millard (1990: 211) concludes that "the concept of scheduled feedings dominates as a consistent, central concern. Despite that today's advice is to breastfeed on demand, the clock continues to occupy a central location." This trend is observed in maternity hospitals in Thailand nowadays and this, as I have suggested earlier, is the result of the medicalization of childbirth in the country. Often, women would be told to feed their infants every three or four hours. A few of the urban and educated women would follow this advice. Pimpilai, an urban woman, breastfed her baby every four hours. She remarked:

> I fed the baby according to my schedules; probably every 4 hours. My cousin who is a nurse told me to do so. She said I must write down when I last fed her; don't just feed the baby whenever the baby wanted it. So, after each feed, the baby had to wait at least 4 hours for the next feed.

Millard (1990: 211) suggests that feeding on schedules force women to pay attention on the clock and advice from professionals and this implies that "their own bodily signals, the behaviour of their infants and other lay women are not to be trusted" in their attempts to breastfeed. But, this attempt may be too costly for mothers. As Rima Apple (1987) notes, this "proper" feeding involves "rigid schedules" and all too often mothers fail to sustain adequate milk supplies. Ann Millard (1990) also points out that feeding on schedules would reduce milk supplies and increase infant hunger. This often discourages women to continue to breastfeed. Not only that, irregular pattern of breastfeeding may also have a real physiological effect (Woolridge, 1995; Dykes, 2005). Not surprisingly, Pimpilai said that her breast milk dried up at the end of her confinement period; one month after birth.

> By the time my *yu duan* [confinement practice] finished, I stopped breastfeeding, as I did not have any more breast milk. Around the 15th or 16th day, I still had some. But, by the end of the month, it was totally dried out. I don't know why it happened like this.

But, many mothers resisted this recommendation. They would feed their infant on demand. As Wasana, an urban poor woman, said:

> I would feed my baby whenever she wanted it. So if she cried I believed she was hungry and I would just put her on my breast. I would not wait for two or three hours like I was told. If the baby was not hungry, it would not cry.

Similarly, Nida, an urban woman, told us that:

> I breastfed as often as the babies wanted it; I did not look at the clock or anything. Whenever the babies cried for it, I put them on my breast straight away.

It is also clear that urban educated women tended to make their own observations about their babies' feeding patterns, rather than following the advice
given by health professionals (cf. Manderson, 1985). In Lenore Manderson's
work with the middle-class Australian women, she found that, initially, the
women would follow health professional's advice precisely, but then they
would modify, behind their doctors' back, to suit their babies and their own
situations. In my study, Darunee, for example, suggested that:

> I observed that it was around two hourly that the baby would cry for milk. At
> first, I did not know, so I followed what the doctor told me to do. For a while, I
> started to observe that the baby started to be hungry every two hours. So, I fed
> her every two hours. I checked the clock, and if two hours had passed, I would
> feed the baby; starting with my milk, then bottle and the baby would then go
> back to sleep.

The women also challenge or resist the advice given by health professionals
by following the advice of their own lay advisers, particularly those of their
family members (Millard, 1990). This is clearly seen in the advice women
received to adhere to traditional diet during the confinement period in order
to ensure sufficient milk supply despite the advice against this by health professionals.

CONCLUDING DISCUSSION

> Breastfeeding practices within a given culture represent the ways in which
> women negotiate and incorporate dominant ideologies and institutional and cul-
> tural norms with the realities of their embodied experiences, personal circum-
> stances and social support systems. (Dykes, 2005: 2283)

Breastfeeding has become an international agenda. Fiona Dykes (2005: 2283)
contends that the pressure on women to breastfeed has become increasingly
pervasive. Internationally prescribed guidelines on breastfeeding proliferate.
The World Health Organization (2002) now sets out its recommendation that
women should exclusively breastfeed their newborn infants for a minimum of
six months. This recommendation has gained credence, and health professionals in particular insist on this to new mothers.

Infant feeding practices, however, continue to relate to the local moral
world. In modernizing societies, as Kathleen Barlow (1985: 137) contends,
infant feeding practices "do not exist in isolation from the cultural and socio-
economic environments in which they occur. They result from beliefs and
values which operate within particular ecological environments and socio-

economic situations." Breastfeeding in any society, as such, is not problem-free either. Each society perceives and deals with problems in culturally specific ways (Millard, 1990). The mothers' choice to breastfeed or not, as Majia Nadesan and Patty Sotirin (1998) contend, "encompasses subtle, but compelling conflicting demands, reflecting some of the tensions and contradictions women face in contemporary society."

Infant feeding practices are indeed contentious issues. As Elizabeth Murphy (1999: 205) writes, mothers' decision to feed their babies "carries considerable moral baggage." Indeed, the findings of my study suggest "infant feeding is a moral minefield." The ways that women can be judged, or judge themselves, is clearly articulated in this study. This is an indication that "mothers are all caught in the cross-currents of complex and sometimes contradictory obligations" (Murphy, 1999: 206). Clearly then, infant feeding decisions are not only about nutrition, but more importantly, are about morality.

Whether the women intend to breast or formula feed, they attempt to construct "an image of themselves as moral members of society" (Murphy, 1999: 191; see Douglas, 1970). Mothers' intention to breastfeed is culturally constructed as an act of a good mother. These women follow the rules knowingly, and hence, were not questioned about their maternal morality or felt the need to justify their intentions. Breastfeeding, Murphy (1999: 204) contends, could be perceived as "evidence of being a good mother who is not only knowledgeable but who is also prepared to act on that knowledge." But, this also holds true for mothers who intend to bottle-feed despite some societal ambivalence about their infant feeding intentions. When a feeding decision is made, a mother knows very well that "her decision is vulnerable to the charge of sanctionable deviance." Hence, she must construct an invention in order to defeat such a charge. As such, women must rely on providing a range of justification for their intentions (Murphy, 1999: 200), as the attempts employed by the women in this study.

It seems clear that the discourse on breastfeeding amongst the Thai women in my study relates to ideals of motherhood. Most often, women refer breast milk to "mother's milk" (*nom mae*). This emphasizes the mother and child relationship ideal. The belief that it is a mother's blood that creates her breast milk and the characteristics of a mother is transferred to her child through breast milk reinforces the interconnection between a mother and her child.

It is clear in my study that both breast- and bottle-feeding mothers see themselves as "knowledgeable rather than ignorant." As in Sarah Earle's study (2000: 327) indicates, both breast- and bottle-feeding mothers definitely know that breastfeeding is best for their infants. Nurit Guttman and Deena Zimmerman (2000) too suggest in their findings that regardless of the infant feeding method they adopted, the women spoke highly of the health benefits of breast-feeding. Most also believed that breastfeeding is something a "good mother" should do. However, regardless of their feeding choices, the actual practice of breastfeeding amongst these women was socially constrained. Mothers who bottle-feed attempt to show that their decisions to bottle-feed, which "superficially, seems irreconcilable with responsible motherhood, is perfectly justified" (Murphy, 1999: 205). Clearly, as Guttman and Zimmerman (2000: 1468) contend, "this does not imply that mothers who do not breastfeed care less about the health of their baby. Formula may simply be accepted as a 'good enough' substitute."

The campaign "Breast is best," Nadesan and Sotirin (1998: 230) suggest, "casts the decision to breast-feed as a dualistic choice between 'good' and 'bad' bodies, images, performances, and policies." "Breast is best" is not only a choice over whether women should breastfeed or not, but also "an injunction to perform culturally authorized gender identities" (see also Sheehan, 2006). In the case of my study, it is the gender identity of women as mothers. In addition, we must be mindful that, as Earle (2000: 328) suggests, women do not necessarily lack knowledge to make decisions about infant feeding, but that "there are other significant factors at play." And in this study, I have shown that there are other significant factors including work and insufficient milk dictate whether women choose to breast- or bottle-feed their infants.

In sum, I have demonstrated the many facets of breastfeeding in Northern Thai society. Whether women breastfeed or not is not a straightforward answer. Indeed, as Fiona Dykes (2005: 2292) concludes:

> Breastfeeding is a complex relationship between mother and baby, the wider family and community. It is a fluid, literally and metaphorically, ever-changing activity influenced by the counterbalancing effects of past events, the daily lived experience and future plans.

NOTE

1. WIC is the Special Supplemental Nutrition Program for Women, Infants and Children (WIC) and is responsible for the improvement of nutritional health of vulnerable mothers and children. WIC provides supplemental foods, infant formula, and advice on infant feeding and health-care referrals for mothers from low-income but diverse groups of mothers (Cricco-Lizza, 2005). In 2000, 37 percent of white women enrolled in WIC clinic, 35% were Hispanic and 22% were black non-Hispanic mothers (Fox et al., 2003).

Chapter Eight

Childrearing and Infant Care: Motherhood, Risk, and Responsibility

ﬡ

Throughout history, mothers who failed to love or nurture their babies were
seen as unnatural, unbalanced, and unsavoury, and women suspected [to]
lacking in maternal warmth suffered the malicious gossip and innuendo of
their neighbours

(Scheper-Hughes, 1987: 6)

INTRODUCTION

I wish to start this chapter by making references to two recent studies on child
care and child health: those of Fikree et al. (2005) and Accorsi et al. (2003).
In Fariyal Fikree and colleagues' study (2005), they examined newborn care
practices in low socio-economic settlements of Karachi, Pakistan, while the
burden of traditional practices on child health in Northern Uganda was investigated in Sandro Accorsi and others' study (2003). In these two studies,
despite their recency and their provision of some understanding of mothers'
behaviours toward the care of their children, the researchers point to the danger or burden of the practices of the local moral world on which the mothers
operate. These studies have given little attention to the subjective experiences
of mothers in relation to their social positions and how they see themselves
as a parent and their difficulties and risk entailed in rearing children within
the social and cultural context of their mothering roles.

There are a few exceptions, however. Unlike most studies on childrearing and
child care, Nancy Scheper-Hughes (1987a) undertakes an interesting study on
mothers' emotional responses to their children's health and conditions in a poor
and changing society of Brazil. Her work is a classic example of the importance
of examining the ways mothers make sense of their children's illnesses which

impact their emotional responses, and hence, the ways they care for their ill children within the context of poverty. Her findings point to the importance of "the social and economic context" of women's lives. The expression of maternal sentiments and the cultural meanings of mother love and child death are constructed within the mothers' "experiences of attachment, separation, and loss." Scheper-Hughes (1987a: 187-188) alerts us to a *luta*, "a unifying metaphor of life, a struggle, between strong and weak, or between weak and weaker still." This culturally constructed concept allows mothers to "explain the necessity of allowing some, especially their very weak—babies to die '*a mingua*,' that is, without attention, care, or protection." She suggests that "maternal thinking and practices are socially produced rather than determined by a psychological script of innate universal emotions." Her study points to "the indignities and inhumanities" that these poor mothers have to make decisions; the decisions that no mothers should have to make. The selective neglect of children, Scheper-Hughes (1987a) argues, needs to be understood as a direct result of the selective neglect of their mothers who have been marginalized due to their poverty. (See also Scheper-Hughes, 1984, 1985, 1988, 1991, 1992 and Nations and Rehbun, 1988).

The work of Sonja Olin Lauritzen (1997) is another exceptional piece. She examines the ways mothers make sense of the illness of their young infants. She theorizes that mothers understand health in relation to a double frame of reference, the bodily and the social, as a cue to tell if their infants are healthy or ill. In their attempts to assess the health of their infants, mothers try to 'read' the bodily signs and reactions in their young babies. Mothers feel many threats in their attempts to raise children and these include threats of abnormality, survival, thriving, and ill health. S. Olin Lauritzen (1997: 436) concludes her findings that "the embodied images of child health are intertwined with the mothers' presentation of themselves as responsible for the health of their children as 'worthy' parents."

In this chapter, I discuss childrearing practices and infant care amongst Northern Thai mothers. In particular, I focus on issues relating to risk and responsibility of mothers in their childrearing practices. I also examine the rituals applying to a newborn infant in Northern Thai society. I shall show that in order for mothers to claim that they are good mothers, they have to be responsible mothers by adhering to the cultural beliefs and practices surrounding the newborn infant. These beliefs and practices tie them with not only their family and their society at large, but also the supernatural world.

RISK, RESPONSIBILITY, AND MOTHERHOOD

According to Anthony Giddens (1991: 123), the social world in contemporary societies is organized within the climate of risk. Elizabeth Murphy (2000:

292), following Giddens (1991), contends that our everyday life is preoccu-
pied with the thought of risk. Many decisions about our behaviour are determined by our preoccupation with possible consequences. Individuals are
urged to control or manage their behaviour as responsible and rational in response to what might happen in the future. But, risk is often embedded in individuals' particular lived experience and at a particular point of time, and can
be varied culturally (Rapp, 1995, 1998). However risk is perceived though,
failure to do so often results in "a charge of irresponsibility," and women may
be seen as immoral or bad mothers. Following on from the previous chapter,
where I discuss the deviance and morality of mothers regarding infant feeding, in this chapter, I examine the ways in which these charges are related to
risk and childrearing and infant care in Northern Thailand.

Following Giddens's conceptual framework of self-identity and modernity
(1991), I contend that mothers live in the risk culture of modernity. In this
condition, Giddens (1991: 123-124) theorises, "for lay actors . . . thinking in
terms of risk and risk assessment is a more or less ever-present exercise . . .
The risk climate is thus unsettling for everyone; no one escapes." Risk assessment has penetrated in many areas in the postmodern world (Giddens,
1991; Beck, 1992; Lupton, 1995; Novas & Rose, 2000; Olin Lauritzen &
Sachs, 2001; Scott et al., 2005; See also chapter 3 in this volume) including
the world of childrearing and infant care (Murphy, 2000). Giddens (1991:
181-182) points out that "radical doubt filters into most aspects of day to day
life," and "feelings of anxiety may become particularly pronounced during
episodes which have a fateful quality when individuals may be forced to con-
front concerns . . . normally [kept] well away from consciousness"; mothers'
concerns with childrearing practices and child care in the early period of their
infants' lives, I suggest, is one such period. Giddens (1991) contends that
once an individual has acknowledged risk, he or she is made to accept that
things can go wrong at any time and any given situation. Giddens further argues, in a situation where the person has "well-established feelings of trust,"
this will not be problematic. However, "if [her] sense of basic trust is fragile,
. . . contemplating a small risk, particularly in relation to a highly cherished
aim," such as ensuring that a child is to thrive, without danger and survive,
"may prove intolerable."

I shall show in this chapter that the mothers' decisions to rear their children
are elaborated upon the modern notion of risk. Risk assessments, according to
Sonja Olin Lauritzen and Lisbeth Sachs (2001: 498), "are pointers to a potential, yet unformed, eventuality." In the case of childrearing and infant care,
the concern may not in itself signify the existence of danger, but may indicate
a future possibility of such adverse events including child illness and death.
As Simon Carter (1995: 135) puts it, "the idea of risk is multifaceted . . . because it simultaneously points to the possibilities of security and insecurity."

In the uncertain world of modernity, risk abounds and creates anxiety for those involved. Anthony Giddens (1991: 182) argues, for most people, knowledge of "high-consequence risks" is "a source of unspecific anxieties." Giddens (1991) theorizes that, modern decisions are constantly bound up in speculation about the future and the control of outcomes. Living in a modern world, the mothers in my study too, wish to control the outcome of their child-rearing and infant care. They become "modern actors," as they are able to "engage in risk assessment," that may point to the well-being or death of future generations (Markens et al, 1999: 367).

Ulrich Beck (1992: 29) suggests that the "catastrophic potential" of a particular event is more important to individuals than the actual statistical probability. According to Beck (1992: 29–30), "no matter how small an accident probability is held, it is too large when one accident means annihilation." Hence, Elizabeth Murphy (2000: 297) argues, "moral accountability" is not counted only on "the magnitude of the risk but also of the value of that put at risk." What mothers do which is seen as attracting potential risk to their infant's health and well-being, even a slight risk, will invite blame.

In the modern world, as Scott and others (2005: 1870) point out, an individual is "at risk" of something, and "the category of 'being at risk' may be said to constitute a new source of social identity" (see also Novas & Rose, 2000). Here, I argue that in relation to childrearing and infant care, the presence of children who are deemed to be 'at risk' has culturally constructed a new identity for women; the identity of women as responsible and moral mothers. Like infant feeding practices, childrearing practices have been bound with "moral judgements" of mothers (Murphy, 2000: 296; Ribbens et al., 2000; see also chapter 7 in this volume). Discourses around childrearing practices, Murphy (2000: 295) contends:

> reflect and reproduce an ideology of motherhood, within which it is mothers who are ultimately held responsible for how children turn out. Mothers' main function is assumed to be maximizing the physical and psychological outcomes for their children and any suggestion that mothers are not energetically pursuing their goal leaves them, at least potentially, vulnerable to criticism.

Motherhood is a moral enterprise (Murphy, 2000: 298). As such, we can anticipate that neglecting to protect the health and well-being of their children "will render mothers morally accountable" (Murphy, 2000: 298; Ribbens et al., 2000; Barnard 2005). Mothers, who ignore certain potential risk reducing such as traditional rituals for newborns, will "find themselves in potential 'moral danger'" (Lupton, 1993: 425). Mothers who fail to ensure the health and well-being of children run the risk of being seen as persons who "failed to act responsibly" (Murphy, 2000: 298). Consequently, mothers' identities as "moral, responsible and prudent persons" (Murphy, 2000: 298) are threatened. I shall show in this chapter that Northern Thai mothers are caught in this cycle of motherhood, risk, and responsibility. And, these mothers set about to do many things in order to establish that they are responsible and good mothers.

GOOD MOTHERHOOD, CHILD HEALTH, AND WELL-BEING: WOMEN'S ACCOUNTS

One of the questions I discussed with the women was that as a mother, what we need to do to make sure that the child will be healthy and well. The way women articulated about being a good mother was essentially related to child health. Most often, mothers referred to the physical health of their newborn and young infants.

> We are mothers, so we need to take good care of our babies. We should give the babies good food, make sure that we feed them so that they are not hungry. If they are hungry, they will cry and would not sleep well. And this is not good for their health. (Malai, a rural woman)

Lakana, a rural woman, also said:

> A good mother must take good care of her baby. She should breastfeed the child when the child cries. She must be careful not to let the child in any sort of danger. If the child has some unusually symptoms like excessive vomit, she must take the child to see a doctor immediately. This is serious and it makes the mother worried.

The emphasis on physical health was also prevalent among urban women. Nida, an urban educated woman, contended:

> Good mothering is to take care of the baby, provide good food, take him to sleep and do not let insects like mosquitoes or ants bite the baby. When the baby can walk, a good mother should make sure that the child won't fall over to hurt himself . . . Well, it is our baby, we love our baby, so we must take the best care for them.

Darunee, an urban educated woman, too suggested that:

> A good mother must pay close attention on her baby. She must provide food, milk and give the baby a bath so that the baby is clean. All these will make the baby healthy and strong.

Poor women in particular emphasized the importance of good health and future life. They remarked that if a mother made sure that the baby was in good health, the baby would have a better future as they would do well with their education. It is not surprising to see this type of remark among poor women. Alaka Basu and Rob Stephenson (2005: 2011) contend that "education . . . has been embraced as the panacea for all ills. Not only is it supposed to drive power, reason and civilization, but in the process it also seems to reduce poverty, unemployment, [and] all the malaise of the contemporary world." Kesara, a rural poor woman, suggested that:

> A good mother must take care of her baby's health, making sure that the baby is warm and has enough clothes to wear and good food to eat. This is the way to ensure that the baby will be healthy, have a good brain to be smart at school.

For urban educated women, they are not only concerned about the physical well-being of their newborn infants, but also the emotional well-being. Pimpilai, an urban woman, had this to say:

> A good mother will give the baby love and warmth. She also needs to make sure that the baby gets good food or food appropriate to her age. She should cuddle her and take good care of her. You can't just feed the baby and then leave the baby by herself. Modern mothers are told not to carry the baby around as the baby will be used to it and then the baby will make demands on the mother. But, I think by carrying the baby around, the baby will receive more love and warmth from the mother. Little babies can feel these things by our touch, so we must touch the baby by carrying the baby with us. As a good mother, we must also talk to the baby even though she might not understand us, but it will be better for the baby if we do so.

Prapaporn, another urban educated woman, told us that:

> A good mother must make sure that the baby is not hungry. She must make sure that her baby is happy and well. She must make the baby comfortable physically and mentally. She must ensure that the baby is not too hot or too cold and because of this the baby will have a good temperament and will then be a happy child.

Urban educated women also talked about being close to their infants as a way to portray good motherhood. Despite the fact that these women had support at home, whether from family members or housemaids with child care, they would still ensure that their infants would fully receive their attention.

> As a good mother, I would look after my own baby; I would do everything for her. When the baby could take it, I would prepare things like mashed rice my-

self. And when I go to work, I take her with me. Hence, I would say that the baby is always close to me. (Patanee)

For some women, who have lost babies through a miscarriage or neonatal death, they would pay a closer attention to their infants. Women felt anxious about the risk of losing another baby. Wilai, an urban educated woman, was one of these mothers and she contended that:

> I must take really good care of the baby. He must be within my sight all the time, even when I went to a bathroom, I would take him with me. I was so afraid that something might happen to him like the one before. I would not take my baby anywhere, even go shopping, because I was afraid that he might catch something.

Good mothers must also knowingly breastfeed their infants (see chapter 7 in this volume). This was not only breastfeeding itself, but also any knowledge regarding breast milk and good infant feeding practices. Any failure on the part of the mothers will elicit blame if the infants become ill. Malai, a rural woman, was unfortunate enough to discard colostrum as she was having pain in her breasts. She squeezed the milk out without realizing that colostrum was also discarded. She was blamed for this.

> The baby did not get the chance to get colostrum because I squeezed it out. I didn't know and I had pain in my breasts, so I squeezed a bit of milk out. My husband was very angry with me because the baby did not get colostrum. The baby was not that healthy; he was ill very often, like every month he would get something. He was hospitalized every month because of his illness. It happened too often; from 7 months to around 3 years old. My husband believed that the baby was like this because he did not get my colostrum. I know that it is the best thing for the baby, but I made a mistake.

Good motherhood goes beyond only knowing about the health and well-being of her infant. This is reflected in women's accounts of infants' cries. When discussing the cry of young children, very often women would comment that as a good mother, one should not let the child cry for too long. The child would only cry when he or she was in need of something, such as being hungry or feeling uncomfortable. A good mother would immediately attend to the child cry and needs (cf. Carrier, 1985). Achsah Carrier (1985: 194) points out in her work with mothers in Ponam, Papua New Guinea that Ponam mothers do not believe infants should be left to cry. These mothers perceived that infants have not yet learned about social and moral responsibility, and it is wrong to force them to learn by being left alone to cry. In fact, these mothers never let the child cry out, they would anticipate and prevent this happening.

In my study, Sangchan, a rural woman, made comments about mothers who left their children to cry too long.

> I would not be able to do that. I would feel sorry for the child; how could his mother leave him to cry like that? When the child cries, it may mean that the child is hungry. I have got a neighbour who left her child to cry like that. She was by herself as her husband was working on a construction site elsewhere. The baby went to sleep and she just went out like that. The baby was crying until he lost his voice and went to sleep due to exhaustion. How could she leave him to cry!

Pimjai, another rural woman, also remarked:

> How could one call oneself a good mother if one leaves the baby cry for too long? What happens if the baby cries too long and he can't stop? He might have a shock and die. This is not a good mother. The baby is ours and if the baby cries we have to console him and take good care of him. It is our baby; it is not easy to become pregnant, give birth and raise him. How could we leave a baby to cry like that!

Nida, an urban educated woman, also said that:

> I would feel sorry for a child who is left to cry by his or her mother. Even though the child is not mine, and even if I would be accused of interfering with them, I would still go in to console him or her. I would not leave him or her to cry like that. A good mother would not do a thing like this?

As in many parts of the world (Ball et al., 1999; Abel et al., 2001; Hooker et al., 2000; Ball, 2002, 2003), bed sharing is a common childrearing practice in Northern Thailand. From birth to about two or three years old, the child will sleep with his or her parents, but very often with the mother. During *yu duan* period, the infant will be placed next to the mother and when the mother moves into her own bed, the infant continues to be near the mother. This practice was seen as essential for the well-being of newborn infants (cf. Morelli et al., 1992; Rice & Naksook, 1998; Ball et al., 1999; Hooker et al., 2000; McKenna, 2000; Abel et al., 2001; Liamputtong, 2001; Ball, 2002, 2003). Mayan mothers in Gilda Morelli and colleagues' study (1992) put their babies with them in their beds, and these mothers asserted that this practice was good for the babies' present needs as well as future development. This practice is a reflection of a good motherhood norm in Mayan culture. As Sally Abel and others (2001: 1140) suggest in their study in New Zealand, "bedsharing was not only a strong cultural tradition for Pacific families but it was perceived to have many . . . psychological and spiritual benefits for the baby . . . It was beneficial psychologically and spiritually in that the baby received love, comfort and moral and spiritual strength by sleeping with its mother." In my study, this is also a reflection of mothers' minds.

> My baby sleeps with me because the baby needs love and warmth from his parents. If the baby is with us, he can feel our bodies, particularly when I cuddle him in bed. I am sure he would receive my love because when I do this in bed, he would look at my face with his innocent eyes. (Darunee, an urban educated woman)

Pimpilai, an urban woman, told us that her newborn baby slept with her and her husband. When asked for the reason, she explained that:

> Because I am worried about the baby. If he sleeps far away from me, he will not feel the warmth from his parents. If he is with us in our bed, we can feel him all the time. I would use my hand to touch his body while sleeping, so that he would not jerk and he would sleep well as he knows that his mother is next to him.

Being close to the infant was also given as reasons for bed sharing. Sirin, an urban educated woman, also said:

> My baby sleeps in the middle between my husband and myself. I want him to be close to me or his parents. When he wakes up, he would know that he is with his mum and dad and I want him to feel like that too.

Malai, a rural woman, had this to say:

> My baby sleeps with me. I was afraid that the baby might be cold. If the baby is close to me then I could cuddle him. He would not be able to stay separate from me. I, as a mother, also want him close to me because I love him and he is my baby. The baby is with me for the whole night.

The practical aspect of bed sharing (Rice & Naksook, 1998; Abel et al., 2001; Liamputtong, 2001; Ball, 2002, 2003) was also perceived by some women in my study who mentioned that having the infant sleep with them was more practical and easy for them with looking after their babies at night time.

> I put the baby to sleep next to me. It is practical for me. At night I don't have to get up to change the nappy or whatsoever and to feed the baby, so it is much more practical and easy when the baby is next to me. Unlike when I was in the hospital, it was so difficult to get up, go to the baby and look after it. It was not practical at all. (Wasana, an urban poor woman)

For some urban educated women, however, they might put the infant on a separate bedding. But, it was still next to their own bed. This was not only for the practical reasons as mentioned above, but they did not want to take risk of smothering the newborn.

> The baby sleeps with me, not on the same bed but on a separate sleeping bedding next to my bed. It is practical for me to feed the baby at night; I just sit up and put her on my breasts. The reason for having a separate bedding is because I am afraid that I might turn my body on top of her and then smother her. (Warunee, an urban educated woman)

RITUALS FOR NEWBORNS IN THE FIRST MONTH OF LIFE: HEALTH, PROSPERITY, AND SAFETY

In any society, cultural beliefs and practices function as a protection and reduce negative outcomes for the societal members including newborn infants. As in other parts of Thailand, Northern Thai people have to perform many rituals for a newborn infant as well as the mother. Most often, the symbolic importance of these rituals is to ensure the health and well-being of the newborn. Here, I discuss several rituals.

Informing *Phi Ban-Phi Heuan* (House Spirits) before Entering a Home

Before bringing a newborn into the house, it is common for almost all women to have a member of the older generation to perform an informing ritual to the house spirit, most often referred to as *phi ban-phi heuan* (but there is a variation of this, sometime they are referred to as *phi heuan-phi ho*, or *chao thi-chao thang*). This is to inform the spirits that there is a new life to be added into the family members and to bless the baby for good health and well-being. When informing the spirits, two incense sticks, a candle, and a bunch of flowers must be placed at the spirit house.

> Before we can take our newborn baby inside the house, we need to inform *phi heuan-phi ho* and the land spirit. We ask blessing for our baby and the mother; let them be happy and healthy and prevent the baby crying at night. We do this and then we do a wrist tying to call the baby's *khwan* in. (Orachorn, a rural woman)

Pimpilai, an urban educated woman, also practised this informing ritual. She stated:

> I inform *chao thi-chao thang* that we now have a new family member and ask them to protect the baby. I ask them to bless the baby with no ill health and to

grow well. I told them that they have got another grandchild in the house and they must protect their grandchild.

Similarly, Prapaporn, another urban educated woman, had this to say:

> My mother told me that before we could bring the baby into our house, we must light the incense stick and candle to inform *chao thi-chao thang* first. It is like we have a new member to be added into the family, *chao thi-chao thang* must be informed so that they will protect the newborn. So, my husband did so before we took our baby into the house when we came back from the hospital.

Rab Khwan: A Wrist Tying Ritual

It is customary in Thailand and Northern Thailand that a *rab khwan* (a wrist tying ritual) is performed for a newborn infant at the end of *yu duan* period (confinement practice; see chapter 5 in this volume). This ritual is a marker of *ok duan* (exit the *yu duan* ritual) of the baby; meaning, like the mother, the baby is no longer bound to the room and house.

Nowadays, as women give birth in hospitals, this ritual might also be done on the day the infant returns home with his or her mother. Essentially, a member of the older generation such as a grandmother or grandfather will be the one who performs a wrist tying ritual. White cotton threads are tied around the wrists of the newborn infant accompanying a blessing such as "let you be with your father and mother; no illness or danger come close to you; let you live well and have plenty to eat," or "let you live well and happy, grow up to have a high status and receive respect from people around you."

A wrist tying ceremony is also a reflection of a strong family member tie within a family lineal in the North. It is said that a deceased family member will be reincarnated into a newborn baby in the family.

> We had a wrist tying ceremony done. It was for welcoming the newborn as another life in the family. We went to consult *po noi* [a novice] who practices astrology to see who was born into the family and *po noi* told us that it was the deceased son of my father who had reincarnated as my baby. My father had to be the person who welcomed the newborn. My father used a white cotton thread to tie the wrist of the baby and then said that he accepted the baby as his grandchild and asked a blessing for the baby's good health and well-being. (Ruchira, a rural woman)

Wilai, an urban educated woman, also elaborated on this:

> My mother did a *rab khwan* ritual for my baby. She used a white cotton thread tied on the baby's wrists. She also used a one baht coin tied with the thread on

the wrists. This is a symbol of blessing for the wealth of the baby. This coin must be kept; not spent on anything.

Informing *Po Kerd, Mae Kerd,* and Well-being

In the North, *po kerd, mae kerd* (birth father, birth mother) is referred to as the father and mother of the person in previous life. Each individual will have his or her *po kerd, mae kerd*. It is believed that *po kerd, mae kerd* would follow the newborn to see how the new parents take care of their babies. Sometimes, if *po kerd, mae kerd* are concerned about the well-being of their previous children, they may wish to take the newborn baby away; meaning the infant will die. Saijai, an urban middle-class woman, explained this to me:

> A newborn baby must have his or her parents in the last life. They have allowed their child to be reborn, they would then come to see them and often they would want to take the baby back. Hence, the new parents will have to inform them that the baby is no longer theirs. The baby is now ours. So, we have to have some words to say to inform them.

The informing ritual must be done at the end of the confinement period. Parents will bring the newborn to a temple, make an offering of food (*sang khathan*) for *po kerd, mae kerd*. But, this can also be done at home. It is known as *tham pithi satuong* by Northern Thai. Essentially, a family member prepares a set of containers with rice, desserts, young (green) coconut, a miniature set of clothes (trousers and blouse), and a small flag (*toong*). The *satuong* set will be placed at the corner of the house compound and a prayer offering the *satuong* and asking *po kerd, mae kerd* to relinquish their previous babies to the new parents (who promise to take good care of their children) will be chanted at that point.

Some women suggested that the new parents must *tham bun* (make merit) for *po kerd, mae kerd* so that *po kerd, mae kerd* will no longer bother the newborn.

> We must *tham bun* for *po kerd, mae kerd* because they will leave the baby for us. The baby is now ours, but we still have to *tham bun* for them as they are also the baby's parents, but in the past life. They are the ones who allow the baby to be born into our family, so we must respect them. Also, if we *tham bun* for them, they will help looking after the baby; they will make sure that baby will not cry excessively, no illness or anything. (Naree, an urban poor woman)

Pimjai, a rural woman, similarly remarked:

Khon boran [older geneneration] said that *po kerd, mae kerd* are the ones who allow us to be reborn. They will protect a newborn baby from any danger and ill health and hence we must *tham bun* for them.

It is strongly believed in Northern Thailand that *po kerd, mae kerd* are part of the "significant others" of an individual's life. They will continue to be concerned about the well-being of and provide protection for the individual. Northern Thai people, hence, continue to make offerings to *po kerd, mae kerd*, particularly during the main religious ceremonies like the Thai New Year (Songkran) and Buddhist Holy Days (which fall in one day per week of the month). This is seen as an essential part of people's lives in the North.

Although we are this mature, we still have our *po kerd, mae kerd* and we must continue to *tham bun* for them. Whenever we go to a temple to offer food for any spirit or angels, we must prepare a food set for *po kerd, mae kerd*. Whatever ceremony you do, you must prepare one set of food for your *po kerd, mae kerd*. They are part of our lives, and hence, we must continue to respect them. (Naree, an urban poor women)

Winnowing Ritual (*Non Kradong*)

Winnowing ritual has survived in the North despite the country undergoing modernity. Essentially, the newborn baby is placed on a winnow and the person who holds the winnow has to stamp his or her feet loudly three times. During the tossing, a chant must be said: "If it is the spirit baby, take it away; if it is the human baby, let it live well, be healthy, happy, and safe." This must be done at the front of the house, particularly at the bottom of the house steps. It must also be done soon after birth. It is said that this is to trade the baby with the spirits. Hence, the spirits would not take the newborn away. Others said that the ritual is to stop the infants jerking which is seen as detrimental to their health and well-being.

Traditionally, we must put the newborn baby on the winnow and then sell it at the front of the house. This is to prevent the child jerking and also crying at night. If people don't do this, the baby will cry excessively at night and it is not good for the well-being of the whole family. This is very strictly adhered to in the North. (Lakana, a rural woman)

Most often too, some books, writing materials, pens and writing pads and needles are also placed under a piece of material that the infant lies on in the winnow. This is to bless the infant with good future as a scholar (books and writing pads) and have a sharp brain (being clever as the sharpness of the needle). The newborn is usually placed in the winnow for at least three days, but some may do it for seven days after birth, starting from the first day of birth. Some would say that the baby must stay in the winnow for the whole confinement period of 30 days. Pimpilai, an urban educated woman, told us that:

> The first day we returned home from hospital, my husband's parents prepared a winnow with some books, writing pads and money and then they put the baby on the winnow. They said the baby will grow up to be a clever and rich boy. The baby slept on the winnow from the first day home for a few days.

Naming Ritual

Women articulated that naming has significant implications for the health and well-being of a newborn infant (cf. Liamputtong, 2000a, c). In the past, parents would consult noble people like Buddhist monks, *po nan* (men who have been monks but now live as lay persons), and astrologers for an "auspicious" name of their newborn infants, and this necessitates the date of birth of the infants. Traditionally, Thai people take circumstances such as hour of the day, day of the month, and month of the year into account when there is a need for conducting rituals in life cycle events and ceremonies. To begin such rituals as weddings and funerals, for example, the most auspicious time has to be selected. It is said that if the time selected is auspicious, things will go smoothly. On the other hand, an inauspicious time results in disaster. This auspicious period is also applicable to a naming ritual

When a baby is born, the moment it comes into the mundane world, as it is traditionally referred to as *tok fak*, must be recorded as the time of birth. The time as well as the date and year of birth will be recorded at the municipality of the town. The *tok fak* detail (time, date and year of birth) will be used to select an auspicious name for a newborn.

> We have to record the time, date and year of birth. When the child is married, or has to undergo any ceremonious, parents must bring this detail to consult a monk or an astrologer in order to look for an auspicious name for the child. This, we believe, will be good for the child, for example, her marriage will last, and she will be successful in whatever she pursues. (Naree, an urban poor woman)

Nowadays, Northern Thai people become more practical with naming. Most often, a father would look for a name in books that is suitable to the child and this is done by examining the date of the birth. Lakana, a rural woman, had this to say when asked about this:

My aunt picked the name of the baby from the lists of names in hospital. She checked the letters of the name to suit the date of birth of my baby. It was OK with her formal name because it was appropriate for her. But, then we gave her a nickname without consulting anyone and the baby cried all night long; it would not stop. We went to see an astrologer and were told that the nickname was not good for our baby. So, we had to change the nickname, and since then the baby was OK. We believed that the first nickname was not auspicious for her.

Nowadays too, some mothers may search further in books for good meanings of names, as this is believed to determine the future of their infants. Malai, a rural woman, when asked how her children received their names, elaborated on this that:

I picked one from books. My husband looked for good ones from the books. We looked through names which are good for the date that the baby was born and then selected a nice one; the one that has a good meaning for our baby.

And Sirin, an urban educated woman, told us that:

My mother picked the names for both of my children. She used the date and time of birth of the babies and picked names which are suitable for my babies. She had to make sure that there would not be any inauspicious letters in the names. She also looked for names with good meanings too. The name of my first daughter is 'Natnaree.' It means a 'female philosopher.' Mum thinks this is the best name and I think it suits her too because I want her to be smart and clever like a philosopher.

Many mothers from rural areas would take the newborn to a local temple for naming. A monk will be asked to examine the birth date and time of the newborn and an auspicious name is chosen. Women remarked that a name given by a monk is more auspicious and ceremonious, and this would be good for the child's health and well-being. My own father took me to see a well-known monk in the area where I was born. My name, Pranee, was chosen, as it was suitable to my character and it has a good meaning; it means "a living creature." When women were asked what would be the consequences of naming their newborns without taking into account their birth date or time, most would say that the child would have ill health and might not thrive well.

I bought a book to look at some names for my baby. My baby was born on Sunday. The book would tell me that a Sunday-born child cannot have certain letters in the name as it is considered as *kalakini* [inauspicious/has bad consequences]. We can't just give any name to the babies as it will impact on their health and well-being. People say that often the baby might be sick or some bad things

might happen to him. I fear bad consequences, so I had to follow older people's
advice. (Darunee, an urban educated woman)

An auspicious name does not only signify the health and well-being, but also
prosperity of the newborn. Pimpilai, an urban educated woman, remarked
that:

I picked my baby's name from a book. I looked at the birth date and time. The
baby was born on Monday morning, I can't use certain letters and vowels on the
name, so I looked at any good names that do not contains those letters. Older
people say that an auspicious name will influence the baby's future and I believe
them. An auspicious name will prevent the baby from ill health and whatever the
baby will do in the future, he will have luck. Some parents do not choose auspicious names for their children and these children are not prosperous; they
can't do well at school and when they are in a trade, they can't make good prof-
its. This is because their names are inauspicious for them.

Some would suggest that if the infant was given a wrong or inauspicious
name, it would cry excessively, or cry for 100 days. To counteract this, parents must give the infant a different name.

I have heard about an infant who cried for 100 days. This is because his parents
did not find an auspicious name for the infant. They had to find another name
for it. It is amazing to see that when the baby was given a new name, it stopped
crying. (Manee, a rural woman)

Orachorn, a rural woman, told us that:

With my first baby, we did not consult anything. We just gave him a name and
he cried a lot, particularly at night. We took him to see a monk at the local temple. The monk did another *su khwan*, tied his wrists, and gave him a new name.
Since then he was fine and he did not cry too often again.

Very often, women remarked that they should prevent this happening by adhering to traditional belief. In other words, women did not wish to take risk
on the unforeseen event (Becker, 1992). Sumalee, an urban woman, had this
to say:

If we do not pay attention to their birth date and time and just give the baby a
name that we like, older people say that it is not good for the baby. The baby
might cry and be unsettled. He might have some problems like ill health or anything. He might not be strong and healthy and we have to change his name. So,
I think we must do this right thing from the beginning to prevent anything happening to the baby.

Similarly, Sinjai, an urban middle-class woman, elaborated on this that:

> It is a traditional belief and we should follow this tradition if we can. I think peo-
> ple in the old days wanted to ensure that an infant would not be in any danger.
> Picking the right name is one of the things which can prevent danger. People
> nowadays might think that is an old belief, but I think if we listen to and follow
> this advice, it does not pose any danger to the baby anyhow, so we should ob-
> serve the tradition.

Women talked about the risk of not following tradition. They expressed their
fears that "bad" consequences might happen to their infants. Hence, they
wished to prevent this happening and eradicated "risk."

> I believe that the baby's name must be auspicious. I am very cautious about this
> and I also fear the consequences. So, I make sure that I strictly follow the tradi-
> tion. What happens if I ignore the tradition and then the baby becomes ill or
> something bad happens to the baby. I have seen some babies who had inauspi-
> cious names and then became very ill and some of them have grown up with lit-
> tle success. I want to prevent this for my baby, so I always follow the traditional
> way of naming. (Wasana, an urban poor woman)

Some women who had infants who were in a special care unit would be particularly cautious about the name of their infants. For these women, the fear
of losing children was great and they would do anything to prevent this happening including giving an auspicious name to their infants. Araya, an urban
woman, had a baby in an incubator for one week due to his suspicious jaundice. Her baby was born on Saturday. According to Thai astrology, a Saturday born child is believed to be a difficult-to-raise child, as Saturday is a
strong day. Hence, her husband would consult an astrologer for the name to
ensure that the infant would be safe.

> My husband got an astrologer to look into the name for our baby. We followed
> the traditional advice because my baby was born on a Saturday which is not a
> good day to be born; it is a strong day. I have to be cautious about this because
> I was afraid of my baby's health. He was so small when he was born and he had
> to be in the incubator because of his jaundice. If he was not born on Saturday,
> we might not be this cautious about his name.

Rural women in particular would remark that parents cannot just give their
children names, as the children will be sickly. Some suggested that this was
because *po kerd* and *mae kerd* (see earlier section) did not approve of the
name that was conveniently selected, and this would result in the child's illness.

My brother named my baby. He was *po nan* and he knew how to pick a good name for my baby by looking at the birth date and time. Older generations are very cautious about this. If the child receives an inauspicious name, it will not live well and will not be happy. Some people might not believe in this and will just name their babies as they wish. As a result, their babies become ill and they have to find a monk or a medium to examine the problem. I have seen cases like this. A neighbour's child was ill and she was told that the name she gave her baby was not suitable to the baby. So, she had to change the baby's name, and the child recovered from illness. (Suriya, a rural poor woman)

Some urban educated women might not really believe in following a naming ritual as such, but would still fear that if they did not do so, there might be some consequences. Siriporn, for example, said that:

Personally, I don't really think that we need to consult people or books with the children's names. We should be able to name our children whatever we like. But, because there are books that we can read and pick the names and these books did suggest some bad consequences of giving a wrong name to the baby, I did follow too. This is just for my peace of mind.

CHILD HEALTH, ILLNESS, AND WELL-BEING: THE ROLE OF MOTHER

In discussing the health and well-being of their infants, mothers had great fears that something would be wrong with their infants. A constant theme running through the women's accounts of child health was the threats of abnormality in their infants (cf. Olin Lauritzen, 1997; Riewpaiboon et al., 2005). Hence, these mothers were cautious about their activities and diet during pregnancy which could potentially contribute to "abnormality" in their children. At birth, the first thing these mothers wished to know was if their newborn infants were physically "normal" (cf. Riewpaiboon et al., 2005).

The first thing I asked a nurse and doctor was if my baby had a complete 32 physical signs. I was so anxious that the baby might not be normal; you know like missing fingers, missing toes, something like that. (Prapaporn, an urban woman)

Although mothers' worries came to an end when the infant was born and they could see that the infants were physically normal, they continued to be concerned about the infants' health. The infants were too thin, perhaps. Did they take enough breast milk? They might be too cold and would catch a cold. These were constant thoughts going through the minds of these mothers.

As a mother, you don't stop worrying about the health and well-being of your babies. I constantly think about this. Even though we are careful about looking after our babies, still, there might be something that makes them sick, like there might be something in the milk or they don't get enough milk to grow well. (Sinjai, an urban woman)

In my interviews with mothers, I often asked them how they knew if their infants were healthy or not. As Sonja Olin Lauritzen (1997: 438) suggests, "mothers base their assessments of health and illness in close day-to-day observations and what they see as their unique, experiential knowledge of their own children" (see also Cunningham-Burley, 1990; Irvine & Cunningham-Burley, 1991). Women used their lived experiences of being a mother to judge their infants' health. Mothers would often look at the bodily signs and reactions in their infants. Some suggested that if the infant could take milk, sleep well after feeding, and was settled (not crying too much), then he or she would be healthy and well. Most often, crying excessively and being unsettled were good indicators of the child's ill health. Sumalee, an urban woman, said:

If the baby is not ill too often and if it seems contented, then this means the baby is healthy and strong.

As Olin Lauritzen (1997: 448) has found in her study, mothers would often compare the health of their child with the health of other children who tended to become ill easily. Some mothers in my study, who had more than one child, would also often compare the conditions of their children as a means to tell about their children's health. Wilai, an urban educated woman, suggested:

As a mother, you can tell. With my first one, I knew he was not strong, but the second is different, he is strong. It is really different. The first one was always sick; he got something most often, you know diarrhea and fever, you name it. He also vomited a lot during feeding. This one is totally different; he eats well, sleeps well, and does not seem to have any ill health.

For some women, the illness of their infants was related to what the mothers did. It might mean that the mother was careless about food or other things, and as a result, this caused some health problem to the child. Mothers blamed themselves for their infants' ill health.

If the child had diarrhea, it must be something to do with the mother. But, I am always careful with food for the baby, so my baby is always okay. (Isara, a rural woman)

Sumalee, an urban woman, said her baby vomited excessively at four months old. She took him to see a doctor and:

> I was told that the baby had a virus in his stomach and it might be because of the food he had. I think I did not clean the bottle properly and so the doctor gave him some medication. Not long afterward, he recovered.

Mothers were cautious about their diet during lactation, as whatever they consumed would get into breast milk and this can make the infant ill. Some mothers who could not breastfeed their infants would give their infants formula milk. To these women, bottle-feeding was not seen as something a bad mother would do. In fact, they were good mothers, who would find food to feed their infants so that the infants might thrive (see chapter 7). As Olin Lauritzen (1997: 446) shows in her study too, one mother attempted to combine breast with bottle-feeding. In response to the advice given by health professionals to continue breastfeeding, she said, "there is all the theory in the world, and that's fine, but unless it's practically working for you it's not fine." She eventually started with breast milk and topped up with infant formula. She believed this filled her baby up and it made her baby happy. The point I want to make is that mothers would do anything to make their infants thrive, and the women in my study were no exception.

In our conversations, I also asked mothers what they did or would do if the child was ill. Very often, mothers would consult family members and friends about the ill health of their infants before seeking care from health professionals. If the illness was seen as minor, pharmaceuticals or simple remedies at home would be the first attempt. Commonly enough, if the baby was diagnosed as having wind in the stomach, which caused a stomach ache, a home remedy was applied. Mothers would use a common household medicine called *mahahing* (a traditional medicine made from an alcoholic substance) to rub on the abdomen of the infant. It is said that *mahahing* would get rid of the pain in the abdomen.

For rural poor women, if the illness was minor such as a cold, they would go to a drug store and buy pharmaceutical products over-the-counter as their first attempt to help the infant or young child (cf. Grace, 1998). If this failed to help the infant, or the condition was serious, mothers would then take the baby to a health center or a hospital. But, for most middle-class women, they would take their infants to see a doctor immediately. Jocelyn Grace (1998) suggests that women who are more educated and come from urban middle-class status are more likely to seek treatment for their children at clinics and health care centers than those from rural and poor mothers. In this study, Sinjai, an urban middle-class woman, told us that:

If the baby cries, it might mean that he is not well. I have to check his condition and then take him to see my doctor straight away. When he was younger, I had to do this very often. If he had a fever, I would be very cautious about him. I was afraid about this as I have heard that if the child has a high temperature, he might have a convulsion and this is very dangerous for a young child. Some might become disabled because of this. So, if the baby had a fever I took him to see a family doctor. I would ring him up and he would see the baby straight away. It is not difficult seeing a doctor, as we live in the town and it only takes a few minutes to get to the doctor.

Again, in Sinjai's case, her financial situation allowed her to seek personal help from her own doctors. Warunee, another urban educated woman, whose child was quite ill, gave her account of her attempt to help her child:

When he was about one year old, he had high fever. I took him to see a local doctor and he told me to give the child paracetamol, but the temperature did not come down; it was just below 40 c. I cooled his body down but it did not help. We were very worried about this because we were afraid that he might have a convulsion due to the fever. I took him to a hospital and begged them to admit my child. I was so afraid of a convulsion and I thought the baby should be close to the doctor.

Of interest was that many women who did not want to risk losing the baby would seek both Western and traditional health care. These mothers adopted what Harold Gould (1965) and Isabelle de Zoysa and others (1984) refer to as "rustic pragmatism"; that is mothers would do anything or try anything that is culturally acceptable in order to make the children survive (cf. Grace, 1998). They would take the children to a clinic or hospital or health center to seek help from modern medicine and at the same time they would also take their children to a temple to be blessed by a Buddhist monk. Some mothers would also seek help from *mor muang* (a traditional herbal healer). This was more marked about rural women; however, some urban mothers did so as well.

At certain times, if modern medicine did not help the infant, a mother would seek traditional health care or consult the spirit medium, referred to as *po mor*. This was also more prevalent among rural poor women. Sangchan, a rural woman, for example, told us that her infant was ill and:

The doctor could not help my baby, so I took him to see *po mor* [spirit medium] to find out what actually happened, as it might be that *po kerd, mae kerd* wanted some thing from us and they made the baby ill. And if it is so, we would have to make *sangkathan* [offering food and clothes] for them, because whatever we did, it would not help the baby. *Po mor* told us that *po kerd, mae kerd* wanted two sets of black and white clothes, and we made the offering to them. We also offered a jar of whisky and a pair of chickens, and the baby recovered from her illness.

What I have presented above is what Jocelyn Grace (1998) and Iftikhar Malik and colleagues (1992) have suggested in their studies in rural Indonesia and Pakistan. Mothers' decisions about where to seek treatment for their infants is made not only on the basis of their socio-economic factors, but also on their understanding of their local moral world, their beliefs in the healers, and the appropriateness of the treatment they provide. In addition, as Sonja Olin Lauritzen (1997: 454) contends, these mothers see themselves as being responsible for their babies' health and well-being. They are the ones who know what is best for their infants (see also Blaxter & Peterson, 1982; Cunningham-Burley & Irvine, 1987; Irvine & Cunningham-Burley, 1991; Mayall & Foster, 1989).

PROHIBITED BEHAVIOURS: INFANTS' SURVIVAL

The mothers' fears about risks which impacted the health and well-being of their infants were expressed in terms of what they **should not do** so that their infants might not be affected by any known and unknown agents. As Olin Lauritzen (1997: 444) contends, this is what mothers see as the threat to the survival of their infants, and this threat is "linked to the ultimate responsibility" that mothers have for the health and well-being of their infants.

All mothers in my study recognized the dangers inherent in childrearing, and they established means to deal with dangers. All mothers made sure that they observed certain traditional practices to ensure the health and well-being of their newborn infants. There are numerous cultural precautions regarding the infant's health and well-being. Some beliefs were observed even before the birth. One important precaution was not to prepare anything for the newborn. Several mothers mentioned that they did not buy anything for their baby. The main reason given was that such preparation can be an inauspicious omen; that is, the infant may die soon after birth if the parents prepare their things for them prior to birth (see also chapter 2).

Most rural poor women observed this cultural precaution, as they believed in the older generation's wisdom and knowledge. Pimjai, a woman from Mae Chantra, did not prepare anything for her newborn baby. This is what she said:

If you are talking about a Northern Thai cultural practice, we cannot prepare anything in advance. People believe that something will happen to the baby if we prepare things for it. The baby will be in danger [die]. I did not prepare any-thing for my baby. When older people tell you anything, you need to believe them and follow their advice. They know better and it is not good for us it we do not follow their advice.

Traditionally, most cultural precautions are observed strictly during the first month after birth, when the mothers observe a confinement practice (*yu duan*—see chapter 5). During the *yu duan* period, parents and significant oth-ers must be cautious about the well-being of the infant. In particular, they must not say good things about the newborn such as "the baby is cute" since the spirits may want to take the infant away with them, or that "the baby is strong and chubby" for fear that the opposite effects of weakness and weight loss may be the result.

> People can't say the baby is cute or beautiful, they must say that the baby is ugly instead. Even a word like heavy, Northern Thai people would not be allowed to say, it is really serious because the baby would become light [meaning thin]. (Is-ara, a rural woman)

Additionally, the infant is not taken outside the house compound until the mother finishes her confinement practice. There are two main reasons for this. First, like the mother, the newborn baby's body is still weak and "cold." If the baby is exposed to outside weather and wind, he or she may become ill easily. Secondly, there are many evil spirits outside the house compound who can harm the infant. As a result, he or she may become seriously ill or die.

> During the first month of life, the baby is still very weak and if we take the baby outside the house compound, spirits may see the baby and it might make the baby sick. Older people would not let us take the baby out. If you walk around the house compound, it is OK, but not outside the house fences. Within the house fences, the spirits of the house would protect the baby, but outside the house fences, there are lots of evil spirits who would make the baby sick and they can take the baby away with them [death of the newborn]. (Naree, an ur-ban poor woman)

CONCLUDING DISCUSSION

Childrearing practices and child care in every society occur in accordance with the cultural norms of the society. In most societies, however, childrear-ing practices and child care share a common value: the preservation of life and maintenance of the health and well-being of a newborn infant (LeVine, 1977, 1980; Castle, 1994; Green et al., 1994; Gethin & Macgregor, 1998; Rice &

Naksook, 1998; Liamputtong Rice, 2000a, c). Childrearing and child care in Northern Thailand is no exception.

Sally Abel and colleagues (2001: 1135) contend that as human beings, the way we take care of our infants and children "is invested with moral value and cultural and personal meaning." In the case of my study, I have suggested that the way Thai women look after their infants is tightly tied with the moral value of motherhood, the cultural meaning of mothers in Thai culture, and their personal meaning of being good and responsible mothers.

As good and responsible mothers, women must ensure that their newborn infants and young children are free of "risk," risk which posts danger on their lives or has ill consequences. As good and responsible mothers, women make sure that the child is healthy and well. They observe cultural beliefs and practices and avoid numerous prohibitions to ensure that their infants will be healthy and well. Clearly, as Abel and others (2001: 1145) suggest, by following certain traditional practices such as naming and informing spirits rituals, mothers can claim that they do not transgress their culturally valued practices. This is a way to avoid any negative impacts on their infants. In this light, they, as mothers, have done something to ensure healthy outcomes for their infants.

The women, as Elizabeth Murphy (2000: 320) contends, construct themselves as "active, responsible, [and] rational" mothers whose duties are to enhance and maintain their infants' health and well-being. They have, in Thomas Osborne's word (1997: 185), been "responsibilised." As we have seen, the women in my study do many things which give them legitimation to place themselves within the discourse of good and responsible mothers.

As Anthony Giddens (1991) and Ulrich Becker (1992) suggest, we are living in the modern world where everything we do is seen as risk and we have our obligation or responsibility to make our attempt to reduce the unforeseen risks. This notion is so pervasive in the world of the mothers in Northern Thailand. The women's narratives clearly show that the ideology of motherhood ties closely with the discourse of risk and responsibility.

> The 'good mother' is one who maximizes physical and psychological outcomes for her child, regardless of personal cost (Murphy, 2000: 292).

Why do Thai mothers seek to continue their cultural beliefs and practices despite the fact that Thai society has become modernized? It is clear from the interviews that this is due to the fact that Thai mothers and their families wish to preserve the life of their newborn infants and maintain their good health and well-being for the rest of their lives so that Thai society can continue to exist. Children are important and essential in any society since they are the future of the society (Jenks, 1982; Giddens, 1991; Inhorn, 1996; Liamputtong, 200a, c). But, it is more than that. Taking a social perspective, Marcia Inhorn (1996) argues that children are important for at least two reasons. First, children are necessary in order to secure the survival of their parents and families. Second, children are needed for the continuation of the society. Inhorn's first theory seems to be applicable to Northern Thai society. In Thai culture, children are necessary for one's well-being, particularly when parents are in old age. Thailand has no social security which provides some types of care for older people as in most Western societies. Aged parents are left to be taken care of by the family. Thai people also believe in *bun khun* of their parents (see chapter 1). This *bun khun* concept has been used as a means for children to care for their aged parents. Without children to look after them, older people would not survive, particularly those who are poor and sick.

In conclusion, throughout this chapter, I have provided readers with the cultural construction of childrearing and infant care in Northern Thai society. Thai mothers observe and practice many socially and culturally acceptable tasks to ensure the health and well-being of their infants. Mothers see themselves as responsible parents and hence follow numerous rules to avoid risks which may pose threats to the health and well-being of their infants. This attempt, I conclude, is used as a means to prove that they are good and moral mothers.

In Trying to Conclude . . . Postscript

I have thus far shown that many of the lived experiences of becoming a mother of Thai women in this study are similar to those of mainstream, Western women in literature, but there are many aspects too that set them apart from their Western counterparts. It is clear that the women in this study travel through profound changes in the process of becoming a mother, from becoming pregnant and giving birth to rearing and caring for their newborn infants. Through the journey of motherhood, the women subject themselves to medical dominance, endure birth and its technology, and attempt to observe the many cultural beliefs and practices to make sure that their infants will thrive and survive. They perform many moral obligations by making sure that their infants are not at risk of any dangers. Many mothers have to perform this amidst poverty and lack of support, although some have better resources to help them through this journey.

Feminist scholars (Oakley, 1980; Thurer, 1994; McMahon, 1995; Hays, 1996; Maushart, 1997; Bhopal, 1998; DiQuinzio, 1999; Liamputtong, 2001, 2006; Manne, 2005) have argued that the journey of motherhood is no easy task. As Ann Oakley (1979, 1980) suggests, becoming a mother is a life crisis for women; it is "a journey into the unknown." Sharon Hays (1996: 32) too argues that mothering is not only "emotionally absorbing but also labor-intensive." As Nancy Chodorow (1978) contends, women do become mothers, but the process of becoming a good mother is often problematic and not without contradictions. And when women have to deal with the double identities of motherhood (McMahon, 1995), as a mother and as a poor woman, the journey is even more problematic and burdensome. As I have shown in this book, the women not only had to struggle with the ideologies of moral motherhood, but they also had to simultaneously cope with their social problems in their everyday lives. The societal expectation that motherhood and mothering is an easy and instinctive part of womanhood is, therefore, contested by the women in my study. Indeed, it confirms that becoming a mother is a very complex matter (Weaver & Ussher, 1997). It is imperative that we understand the social and cultural environments in which women try to mother if we are to provide sensitive care to Thai women who choose to become mothers; a task that was, and still is, essential for the survival of Thai society. But, as in any society, childrearing and child-care perceptions and practices are constantly subject to social, cultural, political, and economic changes. How the Thai mothers in my study in particular, and other Thai women in general, would deal with these changes, remains to be seen.

References

ʔ

Abel, S., J. Park, D. Tippene-Leach, S. Finau, and M. Lennan. "Infant Care Practices in New Zealand: A Cross-Cultural Qualitative Study." *Social Science & Medicine* 53 (2001): 1135–1148.

Accorsi, S., M. Fabiani, N. Ferrarese, R. Iriso, M. Lukwiya, and S. Declich. "The Burden of Traditional Practices, *Ebino* and *Tea-Tea*, on Child Health in Northern Uganda." *Social Science & Medicine* 57 (2003): 2183–2191.

Allsop, J., and L. Mulcahy. "Maintaining Professional Identity: Doctors' Responses to Complaints." *Sociology of Health & Illness* 20 (1998): 802–824.

Alpha Research Co., Ltd. *Pocket Thailand Public Health*, 2nd edition. Bangkok: Alpha Research Co., Ltd, 1997.

American Academy of Pediatrics. "Breastfeeding and the Use of Human Milk." *Pediatrics* 100 (1997): 1035–1039.

Antonis, B. "Motherhood and Mothering." Pp. 55–74 in *Women in Society: Interdisciplinary Essays*, edited by Cambridge University Women's Studies Group. London: Virago, 1981.

Anuman Rajadhon, Phya. *Some Traditions of the Thai and Other Translation of Phya Anuman Rajadhon's Articles on Thai Customs*. Bangkok: Thai Inter-Religious Commission for Developmen and Sathirakoses Nagapradipa Foundation, 1987.

Apple, R. *Mothers and Medicine: A Social History of Infant Feeding, 1890–1950*. Madison: University of Wisconsin Press, 1987.

Armstrong, D. *Political Anatomy of the Body: Medical Knowledge in Britain in the Twentieth Century*. Cambridge, England: Cambridge University Press, 1983.

Armstrong, D. "Foucault and the Sociology of Health and Illness: A Prismatic Reading." Pp. 15–30 in *Foucault, Health and Medicine*, edited by A. Petersen and R. Bunton. London: Routledge, 1997.

Arney, W.R. *Power and the Profession of Obstetrics*. Chicago: Univesity of Chicago Press, 1982.

Bailey, C., R.H. Pain, and J.E. Aarvold. "A 'Give It a Go' Breast-Feeding Culture and Early Cessation Among Low-Income Mothers." *Midwifery* 20 (2004): 240–250.

Ball, H.L. "Reasons to Bed-Share: Why Parents Sleep with Their Infants." *Journal of Reproductive & Infant Psychology* 20 (2002): 207–221.

Ball, H.L. "Breastfeeding, Bed-Sharing, and Infant Sleep." *Birth* 30(3) (2003): 181–188.

Ball, H.L., E. Hooker, and P.J. Kelly. "Where Will the Baby Sleep? Attitudes and Practices of New and Experienced Parents Regarding Co-Sleeping with Their Newborn Infants." *American Anthropologists*, 10 (1999): 143–151.

Bankauskaite, V., and O. Saarelma. "Why Are People Dissatisfied with Medical Care Services in Lithuania? A Qualitative Study Using Responses to Open-Ended Questions." *International Journal for Quality in Health Care* 15(1) (2003): 23–29.

Barlow, K. The Social Context of Infant Feeding in the Murik Lakes of Papua New Guinea. Pp. 137–154 in *Infant Care and Feeding in the South Pacific*, edited by L.B. Marshall. New York: Gordon and Breach Science Publishers, 1985.

Barnard, M. "Discomforting Research: Colliding Moralities and Looking For 'Truth' in a Study of Parental Drug Problems." *Sociology of Health & Illness* 27(1) (2005): 1–19.

Barros, F.C., C.G. Victora, and S.S. Morris. "Caesarean Sections in Brazil." *Lancet* 347 (1996): 839.

Basu, A.M., and R. Stephenson. "Low Levels of Maternal Education and the Proximate Determinants of Childhood Mortality: A Little Learning is Not a Dangerous Thing." *Social Science & Medicine* 60 (2005): 2011–2023.

Bauman, Z. *Postmodern Ethics*. Oxford: Blackwell, 1993.

Beal, A. C., K. Kuhlthau, and J.M. Perrin. "Breastfeeding Advice Given to African American and White Women by Physicians and WIC Counsellors." *Public Health Reports* 118 (2003): 368–376.

Beasley, A., N. Chick, M. Pybus, J. Weber, D. MacKenzie, and D. Dignam. "'I Was Scared I Had Run Out of Milk!' Breastfeeding and Perceptions of Insufficient Milk Among Manawatu Mothers." Pp. 57–74 in *Breastfeeding in New Zealand: Practice, Problems and Policy*, edited by A. Beasley and A. Trlin. Palmerston North: Dunmore Press, 1998.

Beatie, E.A. "Women and Childbirth: Expectation and Satisfaction." *Women's Health Issues* 5 (1995): 40–41.

Beck, U. *Risk Society: Towards a New Modernity*. London: Sage, 1992.

Becker, C.S. *Living and Relating: An Introduction to Phenomenology*. Newbury Park: Sage, 1992.

Belizan, J.M., F. Althabe, F.C. Barros, and S. Alexander. "Rates and Implications of Cesarean Sections in Latin America: Ecological Study." *British Medical Journal* 319 (1999): 1397–1400.

Bhopal, K. "South Asian Women in East London: Motherhood and Social Support." *Women's Studies International Forum* 21 (1998): 485–492.

Blair, A. "Social Class and the Contexualization of Illness Experience." Pp. 27–48 in *Worlds of Illness: Biographical and Cultural Perspectives on Health and Disease*, edited by Alan Radley. London: Routledge, 1993.

Blaxter, M. *Health and Lifestyles*. London: Tavistock/Routledge, 1990.

Blaxter, M., and E. Peterson. *Mothers and Daughters. A Tree-Generational Study of Health Attitudes and Behaviour*. London: Heineman Educational Books, 1982.

Bluff, R., and I. Holloway. "'They Know Best': Women's Perceptions of Midwifery Care during Labour and Childbirth." *Midwifery* 10 (1994): 157–164.

Blum, L.M. "Mothers, Babies and Breastfeeding in Late Capitalist America: The Shifting Contexts of Feminist Theory. *Feminist Studies* 19 (1993): 291–311.

Blum, L.M. *At the Breast: Ideologies of Breastfeeding and Motherhood in the Contemporary United States.* Boston: Beacon Press, 1999.

Blumer, H. *Symbolic Interactionism.* Englewood Cliffs, NJ: Prentice Hall, 1969.

Boonchalaksi, W., and P. Guest. *Prostitution in Thailand.* Nakorn Pathom: Institute of Population and Social Research, Mahidol University, 1994.

Boonmongkon, P., M. Nichter, and J. Pylypa, J. "*Mot Luuk* Problems in Northeast Thailand: Why Women's Own Health Concerns Matter as Much as Disease Rates." *Social Science & Medicine* 53 (2001): 1095–1112.

Boonmongkon, P., M. Nichter, J. Pylypa, N. Sanhajariya, and S. Saitong. "Women's Health in Northeast Thailand: Working at the Interface Between the Local and the Global." Pp. 59–80 in *Women's Health in Mainland Southeast Asia*, edited by Andrea Whittaker. New York: The Haworth Press, Inc, 2002.

Boonwanich, P. "The Study of the Effect of the Duration of the Postnatal Maternal Leave and Other Factors to the Pattern of Breast Feeding among the Civil Servants." *Journal of Provincial Hospital* 12(5) (1993): 9–17 (in Thai).

Boonyoen, D., K. Wongboonsin, V. Tangcharoensathien, and P. Wongboonsin. *Economic Crisis and Effects on Reproductive Health in Thailand.* Bangkok: Chulalongkorn University Institute of Population Studies, 1998.

Bordo, S. "Feminism, Foucault and the Politics of the Body." Pp. 179–202 in *Up against Foucault. Explorations of Some Tensions between Foucault and Feminism*, edited by Caroline Ramazanogl. London: Routledge, 1993.

Boulton, M.G. *On Being a Mother: A Study of Women with Pre-School Children.* London: Tavistock, 1983.

Bourdieu, P. *Outline of a Theory of Practice.* Cambridge: Cambridge University Press, 1977.

Bourdieu, P. *Distinction: A Social Critique of the Judgement of Taste.* London: Routledge, 1984.

Bourdieu, P. *The Logic of Practice.* Cambridge: Polity Press, 1990.

Brent, N.B., B. Redd, and A. Dworetz "Breast-Feeding in a Low-Income Population." *Archives of Pediatrics and Adolescent Medicine* 149 (1995): 798–803.

Brown, E.R. "Public Health in Imperialism: Early Rockefeller Program at Home and Abroad." *American Journal of Public Health* 66(9) (1976): 897–903.

Brown, E.R. *Rockefeller Medicine Men: Medicine and Capitalism in America.* Berkeley: University of California Press, 1979.

Brown, R.E. "Breast-Feeding and Family Planning: A Review of the Relationships between Breast-Feeding and Family Planning." *American Journal of Clinical Nutrition* 35 (1982): 162–171.

Brown, S., J. Lumley, and R. Small. *Reasons to Stay, Reasons to Go: Victorian Women Talk About Early Discharge.* Melbourne: Centre for the Study of Mothers' and Children's Health, 1995.

Brown, S., R. Small, and J. Lumley "Being a 'Good Mother.'" *Journal of Reproductive and Infant Psychology* 15 (1997): 185–200.

Brown, S., R. Small, J. Lumley, and J. Astbury. *Missing Voices: The Experiences of Motherhood*. Melbourne: Oxford University Press, 1994.

Browner, C. H., and N. Press. "The Production of Authoritative Knowledge in American Prenatal Care." *Medical Anthropology Quarterly* 10(2) (1996): 141–156.

Brubaker, R., and P. Cooper. "Beyond 'identity.'" *Theory & Society* 29 (2000): 1–47.

Bruce, J. *Fundamental Elements of the Quality of Care: A Simple Framework*. Working papers No. 1. New York: The Population Council, 1989.

Bruce, J. "Fundamental Elements of the Quality of Care: A Simple Framework." *Studies in Family Planning* 21(2) (1990): 61–91.

Brun, V., and T. Shumacher. *Traditional Herbal Medicine in Northern Thailand*. Bangkok: White Lotus, 1994.

Buxton, K.E., A.C. Gielsen, R.R. Faden, and H.C. Brown. "Women Intending to Breastfeed: Predictors of Early Infant Feeding Experiences." *American Journal of Preventive Medicine* 7 (1991): 101–106.

Cai, W.W., J.S. Marks, C.H.C. Chen, Y.X. Zhuang, L. Morris, and J.R. Harris. "Increased Cesarean Section Rates and Emerging Patterns of Health Insurance in Shanghai, China." *American Journal of Public Health* 88 (1998): 777–780.

Callen, J., and J. Pinelli. "Incidence and Duration of Breastfeeding for Term Infants in Canada, United States, Europe, and Australia: A Literature Review." *Birth* 31(4) (2004): 285–292.

Campero, L., C. Garcia, C. DiAz, O. Ortiz, S. Reynoso, and A. Langer. "'Along I Wouldn't Have Known What to Do': A Qualitative Study on Social Support During Labor and Delivery in Mexico." *Social Science & Medicine* 47(3) (1998): 395–403.

Carrier, A.H. "Infant Care and Family Relations on Ponam Island, Manus Province, Papua New Guinea." Pp. 189–206 in *Infant Care and Feeding in the South Pacific*, edited by Leslie B. Marshall. New York: Gordon and Breach Science Publishers, 1985.

Carter, M. "Husbands and Maternal Health Matters in Rural Guatemala: Wives' Reports on Their Spouses' Involvement in Pregnancy and Birth." *Social Science & Medicine* 55 (2002): 437–450.

Carter, S. "Boundaries of Danger and Uncertainty: An Analysis of the Technological Culture of Risk Assessment." Pp. 133–150 in *Medicine, Health and Risk: Sociological Approach*, edited by Jonathan Gabe. Oxford: Blackwell, 1995.

Castle, S. E. "The (Re)Negotiation of Illness Diagnoses and Responsibility for Child Death in Rural Mali." *Medical Anthropology Quarterly* 8(3) (1994): 314–335.

Castro, A., A. Heimburger, and A. Langer. *Cesarean Sections in Mexico: A Qualitative Study with Women and Health Care Professionals*. Mexico: Population Council Regional Office for Latin America and the Caribbean, Safe Motherhood Committee of Mexico, 1998.

Cheung, N. F. "Chinese Zuo Yeuzi (Sitting in for the First Month of the Postnatal Period) in Scotland." *Midwifery* 13(2) (1997): 55–65.

Chintana, P. *Contraceptive Method Choice in Thailand*. Bangkok: National Statistical Office of the Prime Minister, 1986.

Chodorow, N. *The Reproduction of Mothering: Psychoanalysis and the Sociology of Gender.* Berkeley: University of California Press, 1978.

Chu, C. "Tso Yueh-Tzu (Sitting the Month) in Contemporary Taiwan." Pp. 191–204 in *Maternity and Reproductive Health in Asian Societies*, edited by Pranee Liamputtong Rice and Lenore Manderson. Amsterdam: Harwood Academic Press, 1996.

Coates, M.M., and J. Riordan. "Tides in Breastfeeding Practice." Pp. 3–29 in *Breastfeeding and Human Lactation*, 3rd edition, edited by Jan Riordan. Boston: Jones and Bartlett Publishers, 2005.

Cohen, P., and G. Wijeyewardene. "Introduction, in Spirit Cults and the Position of Women in Northern Thailand." *Mankind Special Issue* 14(4) (1984): 249–263.

Cohen, P.T. "The Politics of Primary Health Care in Thailand, With Special Reference to Non-Government Organizations." Pp. 159–176 in *The Political Economy of Primary Health Care in Southeast Asia*, edited by Paul T. Cohen and John Purcal. Canberra: Australian Development Studies Network, ASEAN Training Centre for Primary Health Care Development, 1989.

Collins, P.H. "Shifting the Center: Race, Class, and Feminist Theorizing about Motherhood." Pp. 45–65 in *Mothering: Ideology, Experience, and Agency*, edited by Evelyn N. Glenn, Grace Chang, and Linda R. Forcey. New York: Routledge, 1994.

Conton, L. "Social, Economic and Ecological Parameters of Infant Feeding in Usino, Papua New Guinea." Pp. 97–120 in *Infant Care and Feeding in the South Pacific*, edited by Leslie B. Marshall. New York: Gordon and Breach, 1985.

Cosminsky, S. "Childbirth and Change: A Guatemalan Study." Pp. 205–229 in *Ethnography of Fertility and Birth*, edited by Carol MacCormack. London: Academic Press, 1982.

Cricco-Lizza, R. "Infant Feeding Beliefs and Experiences of Black Women Enrolled in a New York Metropolitan Area WIC Clinic." *Qualitative Health Research* 14 (2004): 1197–1210.

Cricco-Lizza, R. "The Milk of Human Kindness: Environmental and Human Interactions in a WIC Clinic that Influence Infant-Feeding Decisions of Black Women." *Qualitative Health Research* 15(4) (2005): 525–538.

Croghan, R. "First-Time Mothers' Accounts of Inequality in the Division of Labour." *Feminism and Psychology* 1 (1990): 221–246.

Cunningham, A., D.B. Jelliffe, and E.F. Jellife. *Breastfeeding and Health in the 1980s.* New Jersey: Prentice-Hall, Inc, 1991.

Cunningham, J.D. "Experiences of Australian Mothers Who Gave Birth Either at Home, At a Birth Centre, or In Hospital Labour Wards." *Social Science & Medicine* 36(4) (1993): 475–483.

Cunningham-Burley, S. "Mothers' Beliefs About and Perceptions of Their Children's Illnesses." Pp. 85–109 in *Readings in Medical Sociology*, edited by Sarah Cunningham-Burley and Neil McKeganey. London: Tavistock/Routledge, 1990.

Cunningham-Burley, S., and S. Irvine. "And Have You Done Anything So Far?: An Examination of Lay Treatment of Children's Symptoms." *British Journal of General practice* 295 (1987): 700–702.

Cuttini, M., M.D. Santo, K. Kaldor, C. Pavan, C. Rissian, and C. Tonchelia. "Rooming-In, Breastfeeding and Mothers' Satisfaction in an Italian Nursery." *Journal of Reproductive and Infant Psychology* 13 (1995): 41–46.

Davies, D. "Introduction: Raising the Issues." Pp. 1–9 in *Rites of Passage*, edited by Jean Holm. London: Pinter Publishers, 1994.

Davis, R. "Tolerance and Intolerance of Ambiguity in Northern Thai Myth and Ritual." *Ethnology* 13 (1974): 7–24.

Davis-Floyd, R.E. *Birth as an American Rite of Passage*. Berkeley: University of California Press, 1992.

Davis-Floyd, R.E. "The Technocratic Body: American Childbirth as Cultural Expression." *Social Science & Medicine* 38(8) (1994): 1125–1140.

Davis-Floyd, R.E., and C.F. Sargent, eds. *Childbirth and Authoritative Knowledge: Cross-Cultural Perspectives*. Berkeley: University of California Press, 1997.

De Muylder, X. "Caesarean Sections in Developing Countries: Some Considerations." *Health Policy & Planning* 8(2) (1993): 101–112.

De Zoysa, I., D. Carson, R. Feachem, B. Kirkwood, E. Lindsay-Smith, and R. Loewenson. "Perceptions of Childhood Diarrhoea and Its Treatment in Rural Zimbabwe." *Social Science & Medicine* 19(7) (1984): 727–734.

Denny, E. "Liberation or Oppression? Radical Feminism and in Vitro Fertilization." *Sociology of Health & Illness* 16 (1994): 62–80.

Denny, E. "New Reproductive Technologies: The Views of Women Undergoing Treatment." Pp. 207–227 in *Modern Medicine: Lay Perspectives and Experiences*, edited by Simon J. Williams and Michael Calnan. London: UCL Press, 1996.

Dettwyler, K.A. "A Time to Wean: The Hominid Blueprint for the Natural Age of Weaning in Modern Human Population." Pp. 39–72 in *Breastfeeding: Biocultural Perspectives*, edited by Patricia Stuart-Macadam and Katherine A. Dettwyler. New York: Aldine De Gruyter, 1995.

Dettwyler, K.A. "Breastfeeding and Weaning in Mali: Cultural Context and Hard Data." *Social Science & Medicine* 24 (1987): 633–643.

DiMatteo, M.R. "The Physician-Patient Relationship: Effects on the Quality of Health Care." *Clinical Obstetric Gynecology* 37 (1994): 149–161.

Dingwall, R. *Aspects of Illness*. London: Martin Robertson, 1976.

DiQuinzio, P. *The Impossibility of Motherhood: Feminism, Individualism, and the Problem of Mothering*. New York: Routledge, 1999.

Donaldson, P.J. "Foreign Intervention in Medical Education: A Case Study of the Rockefeller Foundation's Involvement in a Thai Medical School." Pp. 107–126 in *Imperialism, Health and Medicine*, edited by Vincente Navarro. New York: Pluto Press, 1982.

Douglas, J.D. "Deviance and Responsibility: The Social Construction of Moral Meanings." Pp. 3–30 in *Deviance and Responsibility: The Social Construction of Moral Meanings*, edited by Jack D. Douglas. New York: Basic Books, 1970.

Douglas, M. "Risk As a Forensic Resource." *Daedalus* 119 (1990): 177–191.

Duden, B. *Disembodying Women: Perspectives on Pregnancy and the Uunborn*. London: Harvard University Press, 1993.

Duncan, S., R. Edwards, and T. Reynolds. "Motherhood, Paid Work and Partnering: Values and Theories." *Work, Employment & Society* 17(2) (2003): 309–330.

Durongdej, S. *An Innovation Approach on Promotion of Breastfeeding in Urban Communities.* Bangkok: Department of Nutrition, Faculty of Public Health, Mahidol University, 1991.

Dykes, F. "Western Marketing and Medicine-Construction of an Insufficient Milk Syndrome." *Health Care for Women International* 23(5) (2002): 492–502.

Dykes, F. "'Supply' and 'Demand': Breastfeeding as Labour." *Social Science & Medicine* 60 (2005): 2283–2293.

Dykes, F., and C. Williams. "'Falling by the Wayside': A Phenomological Exploration of Perceived Breast Milk Inadequacy in Lactating Women." *Midwifery* 15(4) (1999): 232–246.

Earle, S. "Why Some Women Do Not Breast Feed: Bottle Feeding and Father's Role." *Midwifery* 16 (2000): 323–330.

Eckhardt, K.W., and G.E. Hendershot. "Analysis of the Reversal in Breast Feeding Trends in the Early 1970s." *Public Health Reports* 99 (1984): 410–414.

Ehrenreich, B., and D. English. *For Her Own Good: 150 Years of the Experts' Advice to Women.* New York: Anchor Press, 1978.

Ehrenreich, B., and A.R. Hochschild. *Global Women.* London: Granta, 2003.

Enger, S.M., R.K. Ross, and L. Bernstein. "Breastfeeding History, Pregnancy Experience and Risk of Breast Cancer." *British Journal of Cancer* 76(1) (1997): 118–123.

Family Health Division. *A Study of Breastfeeding Situation.* Bangkok: Family Health Division, Ministry of Public Health, Thailand, 1994.

Feldstein, R. *Motherhood in Black and White: Race and Sex in American Liberalism, 1930–1965.* Ithaca: Cornell University Press, 2000.

Fernandez, M. E., and B. M. Popkin. "Prelacteal Feeding Patterns in the Philippines." *Ecology of Food and Nutrition* 21 (1988): 303–314.

Fikree, F.F., T.S. Ali, J.M. Durocher, and M. Hossein Rahbar. "Newborn Care Practices in Low Socioeconomic Settlements of Karachi, Pakistan." *Social Science & Medicine* 60 (2005): 911–921.

Fishman, C., R. Evans, and E. Jenks. "Warm Bodies, Cool Milk: Conflicts in Post Partum Food Choice for Indochinese Women in California." *Social Science & Medicine* 11 (1988): 1125–1132.

Fongkaew, W. "Gender Socialization and Female Sexuality in Northern Thailand." Pp. 147–164 in *Coming of Age in South and Southeast Asia: Youth, Courtship and Sexuality,* edited by Lenore Manderson and Pranee Liamputtong. Surrey: Curzon, 2002.

Foster, F., D. Lader, and S. Cheesbrough. *Infant Feeding 1995.* London: The Stationery Office, 1997.

Foucault, M. *The Birth of the Clinic. An Archaeology of Medical Perception.* London: Tavistock, 1973.

Foucault, M. "The Politics of Health in the Eighteenth Century." Pp. 166–180 in *Power/Knowledge. Selected Interviews and Other Writings, 1972–1977,* edited by Colin Gordon. Brighton: The Harvest Press, 1980.

Fox, H.B., M.A. McManus, and H.J. Schmidt. *WIC Reauthorization: Opportunities for Improving the Nutritional Status of Women, Infants, and Children.* Washington, DC: National Health Policy Forum, George Washington University, 2003. Internet Access: http://www.nhpf.org/pdfs_bp/BP_WIC2_8–03.pdf.

Gabriel, A., K.R. Gabriel, and R. Lawrence. "Cultural Values and Biomedical Knowledge: Choices in Infant Feeding." *Social Science & Medicine* 23(5) (1986): 501–509.

Galtry, J. "The Impact on Breastfeeding of Labour Market Policy and Practice in Ireland, Sweden and the USA." *Social Science & Medicine* 57 (2003): 167–177.

Georges, E. "Fetal Ultrasound Imaging and the Production of Authoritative Knowledge in Greece." Pp. 91–112 in *Childbirth and Authoritative Knowledge: Cross-Cultural Perspectives*, edited by Robbie Davis-Floyd and Carolyn F. Sargent. Berkeley: University of California Press, 1997.

Gerrard, J.W. "Breast-Feeding: Second Thoughts." *Pediatrics* 54 (1974): 757–764.

Gethin, A., and B. Macgregor. "Cry Baby, Cry." *Melbourne's Baby* July (1998): 8–9.

Giddens, A. *Modernity and Self-Identity: Self and Society in the Late Modern Age.* Standford, CA: Standford University Press, 1991.

Gilbert, T. "Towards a Politics of Trust." *Journal of Advanced Nursing* 27 (1998): 1010–1016.

Gilligan, C. *In a Different Voice.* Cambridge, MA: Harvard University Press, 1982.

Gilson, L. "Trust and Health Care as a Social Institution." *Social Science and Medicine* 56(67) (2003): 1452–68.

Ginsburg, F.D., and R. Rapp. "Introduction: Conceiving the New World Order." Pp. 1–17 in *Conceiving the New World Order: The Global Politics of Reproduction*, edited by Faye D. Ginsburg and Rayna Rapp. Berkeley: University of California Press, 1995.

Giugliani, E.R.J., W.T. Caiaffa, J. Vogelhut, F.R. Witter, and J.A. Perman. "Effect of Breastfeeding Support from Different Sources on Mothers' Decisions to Breastfeed." *Journal of Human Lactation* 10 (1994): 157–161.

Glass, J., and V. Camarigg. "Gender, Parenthood, and Job-Family Compatibility." *American Journal of Sociology* 98 (1992): 131–151.

Glei, D.A., and N. Goldman. "Understanding Ethnic Variation in Pregnancy-Related Care in Rural Guatemala." *Ethnicity & Health* 5(1) (2000): 5–22.

Glenn, E.N. "Social Construction of Mothering: A Thematic Overview." Pp. 1–29 in *Motherhood: Ideology, Experience and Agency*, edited by Evelyn N. Glenn, Grace Chang, and Linda R. Forcey. New York: Routledge, 1994.

Goffman, E. *Asylums: Essays on the Social Situation of Mental Patients and Other Inmates.* Harmondsworth, Middlesex: Penguin Books, 1961.

Goffman, E. *Stigma: Notes on the Management of Spoiled Identity.* Englewood Cliffs, NJ: Prentice Hall, 1963.

Goldsmith, J. *Childbirth Wisdom From the World's Oldest Societies.* Brookline, MA: East West Health Books, 1990.

Golomb, L. *An Anthropology of Curing in Multiethnic Thailand.* Urbana: University of Illinois Press, 1985.

Gonzalez, R. "A Large Scale Rooming-In Program in a Developing Country: Proceeding of the Interagency Workshop on Health Care Practices Related to Breastfeeding." *International Journal of Gynaecology and Obstetrics* 31 (1990): 1–5.

Gould, H.A. "Modern Medicine and Folk Cognition in Rural India." *Human Organization* 24 (1965): 201.

Gould, J.B., B. Davey, and R.S. Stafford. "Socioeconomic Differences in Rates of Cesarean Section." *New England Journal of Medicine* 321 (1989): 233–239.

Grace, J. "The Treatment of Infants and Young Children Suffering Respiratory Tract Infection and Diarrhoeal Disease in a Rural Community in Southeast Indonesia." *Social Science & Medicine* 46(10) (1998): 1291–1302.

Gray, B. "Trust and Trustworthy Care in the Managed Care Era." *Health Affairs* 16 (1997): 34–49.

Gray, R., O.M. Campbell, R. Apelo, S.S. Eslami, R.M. Ramos, J.C. Gehert, and M.H. Labbok, M.H. "The Risk of Ovulation During Lactation." *Lancet* 335 (1990): 25–27.

Green, E.C., A. Jurg, A. Djedje. "The Snake in the Stomoch: Child Diarrhea in Central Mozambique." *Medical Anthropology Quarterly* 8(1) (1994): 4–24.

Greiner, T., P. Van Esterik, and M. Latham. "The Insufficient Milk Syndrome: An Alternative Explanation." *Medical Anthropology* 5 (1981): 233–247.

Grossman, L.K., J.B. Larsen-Alexander, S.M. Fitzsimmons, and L. Cordero, L. "Breastfeeding among Low-Income, High Risk Women." *Clinical Pediatrics* 28 (1989): 38–42.

Gubrium, J.F., and J.A. Holstein, eds. *Handbook of Interview Research*. Thousand Oaks, CA: Sage Publications, 2001.

Gunnlaugsson, G., and J. Einarsdottir. "Colostrum and Ideas about Bad Milk: A Case Study From Guinea-Bissau." *Social Science & Medicine* 36 1993): 283–288.

Gussler, J.D., and L.H. Briesemeister. "The Insufficient Milk Syndrome: A Biocultural Explanation." *Medical Anthropology* 4 (1980): 145–174.

Guttman, N., and D.R. Zimmerman. "Low-Income Mothers' Views on Breastfeeding." *Social Science & Medicine* 50 (2000): 1457–1473.

Hamlyn, B., S. Brooker, K. Oleinikova, and S. Wands. *Infant Feeding 2000*. London: The Stationary Office (TSO), 2002.

Hanks, J.R. *Maternity and Its Rituals in Bang Chan*. Ithaca: Cornell Thailand Project, Cornell University Press, 1963.

Hanvoravongchai, P., J. Letiendumrong, Y. Teerawattananon, and V. Tancharoensathien. "Implications of Private Practice in Public Hospitals on the Cesarean Section Rate in Thailand." *Human Resources for Health Development Journal (HRDJ)* 4(1) (2000): 1–12.

Harley, D. "From Providence to Nature: The Moral Theology and Godly Practice of Maternal Breastfeeding in Stuart England." *Bulletin of Historical Medicine* 69 (1995): 198–223.

Hays, S. *The Cultural Contradictions of Motherhood*. New Haven: Yale University Press, 1996.

Hill, P.D. "The Enigma of Insufficient Milk Supply." *American Journal of Maternal and Child Nursing* 16(6) (1991): 312–316.

Hillervik-Lindquist, C. "Studies on Perceived Milk Insufficiency: A Prospective Study in a Group of Swedish Women." *Acta Pediatrica Scandinavica* 376 (1991): 6–25.

Hills-Bonczyk, S.G., M.D. Avery, K. Savik, S. Potter, and L.J. Duckett. "Women's Experiences with Combining Breast-Feeding and Employment." *Journal of Nurse Midwifery* 38(5) (1993): 257–266.

Holroyd, E., L. Yin-King, L.W. Pui-Yuk, F.Y. Kwok-Hong, and B.L. Shuk-Lin. "Hong Kong Chinese Women's Perception of Support from Midwives During Labour." *Midwifery* 13 (1997): 66–72.

Hooker, E., H.L. Ball, and P.J. Kelly. "Sleeping Like a Baby: Attitudes and Experiences of Co-Sleeping in the Northeast of England." *Medical Anthropology* 19 (2000): 203–222.

Hopkins, K. "Are Brazilian Women Really Choosing to Deliver by Cesarean?" *Social Science & Medicine* 51 (2000): 725–740.

Howell, R.R., F.H. Moriss, and L.K. Pickering. *Human Milk in Infant Nutrition and Health*. Springfield IL: Charles Thomas, 1986.

Hull, V., S. Thapa, and H. Pratomo. "Breast-Feeding in the Modern Health Sector in Indonesia: The Mother's Perspective." *Social Science & Medicine* 30(5) (1990): 625–633.

Hung, B.K., L. Ling, and S.G. Ong. "Sources of Influence on Infant Feeding Practices in Hong Kong." *Social Science & Medicine* 20 (1985): 1143–1150.

Hurst, M., and P.S. Summey. "Childbirth and Social Class: The Case of Cesarean Delivery." *Social Science & Medicine* 18(8) (1984): 621–631.

Ingram, J., and D. Johnson "A Feasibility Study of an Intervention to Enhance Family Support for Breast Feeding in a Deprived Area in Bristol, UK." *Midwifery* 20 (2004): 367–379.

Inhorn, M.C. *Infertility and Patriarchy: The Cultural Politics of Gender and Family Life in Egypt*. Philadelphia: University of Pennsylvania Press, 1996.

Institute of Medicine. *Nutrition During Lactation*. Washington, D.C.: National Academy Press, 1991.

Introduction to Lanna. http://www.chiangmai1.com/chiang_mai/history_3.shtml.(Accessed December 20, 2004).

Irvine, S., and S. Cunningham-Burley. "Mothers' Concepts of Normality, Behavioural Change and Illness in Their Children." *British Journal of General Practice* 41 (1991): 371–374.

Jackson, D.A., S.M. Imong, L. Wongsawasdi, A. Silprasert, S., Preunglampoo, P. Leelapat, R.F. Drewett, K. Amatayakul, and J.D. Baum. "Weaning Practices and Breast-Feeding Duration in Northern Thailand." *British Journal of Nutrition* 67(2) (1992): 149–164.

Jackson, E.B. "General Reactions of Mothers and Nurses to Rooming-In." *American Jouranl of Public Health* 38 (1948): 689–695.

Jackson, E.B. "The Development of Rooming-In at Yale." *Journal of Biology and Medicine* 25 (1953): 486–494.

Jacobson, S.W., J.L. Jacobson, and K.F. Frye. "Incidence and Correlates of Breast-feeding in Socio-Economically Disadvantaged Women." *Pediatrics* 88 (1991): 728–736.

Jamrozik, A., C. Bland, and R. Urquhart. *Social Change and Cultural Transformation in Australia*. Melbourne: Cambridge University Press, 1995.

Jeffery, P., R. Jeffery, and A. Lyon. *Labour Pains and Labour Power: Women and Childbearing in India*. London: Zed Books, 1988.

Jelliffe, D.B., and E.E.P. Jelliffe. *Human Milk in the Modern World*. Oxford: Oxford University Press, 1978.

Jenks, C. *The Sociology of Childhood*. London: Batsford, 1982.

Jirojwong, S. "Health Beliefs and the Use of Antenatal Care Among Pregnant Women in Southern Thailand." Pp. 61–82 in *Maternity and Reproductive Health in Asian Societies*, edited by Pranee Liamputtong Rice and Lenore Manderson. Amsterdam: Harwood Academic Publishers, 1996.

Johnson, M., J. Smith, S. Haddad, J. Walker, and A. Wong. "Women Prefer Hospital Births (letter)." *British Medical Journal* 305 (1992): 255.

Jordan, B. *Birth in Four Cultures: A Crosscultural Investigation of Childbirth in Yucatan, Holland, Sweden, and the United States*, 4th edition. Prospect Heights, IL: Waveland Press Inc, 1997.

Jordan, B., and S. Irwin."A Close Encounter with a Court-Ordered Cesarean Section: A Case of Differing Realities." Pp. 185–199 in *Case Studies in Medical Anthropology: A Teaching and Reference Source*, edited by Baer Hans. New York: Gordon and Breach, 1987.

Kabakian-Khasholian, T., O. Campbell, M. Shediac-Rizkallah, and F. Ghorayeb. "Women's Experiences of Maternity Care: Satisfaction or Passivity?" *Social Science & Medicine* 51 (2000): 103–113.

Kanchanasuk, V., and K. Charoensri. "Socio-Economic and Cultural Change and Women Development." Pp. 1–18 in *Perspective Policies and Planning for the Development of Women*, edited by The National Commission on Women's Affairs [NCWA]. Bangkok: the National Commission on Women's Affairs, 1995.

Kanshana, S. "Maternal Mortality. Fact Sheet—Health Promotion", 1(2) (November, 1–3, 1997). http://www.anamai.moph.go.th/factsheet/health1–2_en.htm.

Kaufert, P., and J. O'Neil. "Analysis of Dialogue on Risks in Childbirth: Clinicians, Epidemiologists, and Inuit Women." Pp. 32–55 in *Knowledge, Power, and Practice: The Anthropology of Medicine in Everyday Life*, edited by Shirley Lindenbaum and Magaret Lock. Berkeley: University of California Press, 1993.

Kay, M. A., ed., *Anthropology of Human Birth*. Philadelphia: F. A. Davis Company, 1982.

Kempe, A., F. Stangard, F. Hamman, F.A. Nooraldin, S. Al Atlas, F.S., Khider, and Z.J. Dhman. *The Quality of Maternal and Neonatal Health Services in Yemen: Seen Through Women's Eyes*. Stockholm: Swedish Safe the Children (Radda Barnen), 1994.

Kerdhet, B. *Status of Thai Women Reflected in Ratanakosin Literature, 1782–1851*. Bangkok: Srinakarinwiroth University, 1974.

Keyes, C.F. "The Northeastern Thai Village: Stable Order and Changing World." *Journal of the Siam Society* 63 (1975): 177–207.

Keyes, C.F. "Mother or Mistress but Never Be a Monk: Buddhist Notions of Female Gender in Rural Thailand." *American Ethnologist* 11(2) (1984): 223–241.

King, J., and A. Ashworth. "Historical Review of the Changing Pattern of Infant Feeding in Developing Countries: The Case of Malaysia, the Caribbean, Nigeria and Zaire." *Social Science & Medicine* 25 (1987): 1307–1320.

Kirsch, V. "Buddhism, Sex-Roles and the Thai Economy." Pp. 16–41 in *Women of Southeast Asia*, edited by Penny Van Esterik. Occasional paper #9. Dekalb: Northern Illinois University, Centre for Southeast Asian Studies, 1982.

Kistin, N., D. Benton, S. Rao, and M. Sullivan. "Breastfeeding Rates Among Black Urban Low-Income Women: Effect of Prenatal Education." *Pediatrics* 86(5) (1990): 741–746.

Kitzinger, S. "The Social Context of Birth: Some Comparisons Between Childbirth in Jamaica and Britain." Pp. 181–205 in *Ethnography of Fertility and Birth*, edited by Carol P. MacCormack. London: Academic Press, 1982.

Kleinman, A. *Patients and Healers in the Context of Culture: An Exploration of the Borderland between Anthropology, Medicine and Psychiatry.* Berkeley: University of California Press, 1980.

Kleinman, A. "Pain and Resistance: The Delegitimation and Relegitimation of Local Worlds." Pp. 169–197 in *Pain as Human Experience: An Anthropological Perspective*, edited by Mary-Jo DelVecchio, Paul E. Brodwin, Byron Good, and Arthur Kleinman. Berkeley: University of California Press, 1992.

Knodel, J. and V. Prachuabmoh. "Desired Family Size in Thailand: Are the Responses Meaningful?" *Demography* 10(4) (1973): 619–637.

Knodel, J., N. Chayovan, and K. Wongboonsin. "Breast-Feeding Trends, Patterns and Policies in Thailand." *Asia-Pacific Population Journal* 5(1) (1990): 135–150.

Kurinu, N., P.H. Shiono, S.F. Ezrine, and G.G. Rhoads. "Does Maternal Employment Affect Breast-Feeding?" *American Journal of Public Health* 79(9) (1989): 1247–1250.

Laderman, C. *Wives and Midwives: Childbirth and Nutrition in Rural Malaysia.* Berkeley: University of California Press, 1987.

Laderman, C. "Food Ideology and Eating Behavior: Contributions from Malay Studies." *Social Science & Medicine* 19(5) (1984): 547–559.

Lane, K. "The Medical Model of the Body as a Site of Risk: A Case Study of Childbirth." In *Medicine, Health and Risk: Sociological Approach*, edited by Jonathan Gabe, 53–72. Oxford: Blackwell, 1995.

Lawrence, R. "The Clinician's Role in Teaching Proper Infant Feeding Techniques." *The Journal of Paediatrics* 126 (suppl) (1995): 112–117.

Lazarus, E. S. "Poor Women, Poor Outcomes: Social Class and Reproductive Health." Pp. 39–54 in *Childbirth in America: Anthropological Perspectives*, edited by Kay L. Michaelson. South Hadley, MA: Bergin & Garvey, 1988.

Lazarus, E.S. "What Do Women Want? Issues of Choice, Control, and Class in Pregnancy and Childbirth." *Medical Anthropology Quarterly* 8(1) (1994): 25–46.

Lee, L.Y.K., E. Holroyd, and C.Y. Ng. "Exploring Factors Influencing Chinese Women's Decision to Have Elective Caesarean Surgery." *Midwifery* 17 (2001): 314–322.

Lee, R. L. "Comparative Studies of Health Care Systems." *Social Science & Medicine* 16 (1982): 629–642.

Lefkarites, M.P. "The Sociocultural Implications of Modernizing Childbirth among Greek Women on the Island of Rhodes." *Medical Anthropology* 13 (1992): 385–412.

Lerdmaleewong, M., and C. Francis. "Abortion in Thailand: A Feminist Perspective." *Journal of Buddhist Ethics* 5 (1998): 22–48.

Leung, G.M., T-H. Lam, T.Q. Thach, S. Wan, and L-M. Ho. "Rates of Cesarean Births in Hong Kong: 1987–1999." *Birth* 28(3) (2001): 166–172.

LeVine, R. "Child Rearing as Cultural Adaptation." Pp. 15–27 in *Culture and Infancy*, edited by Herbert Leiderman, Stephen Tulkin and Anne Rosenfeld. New York: Academic Press, 1977.

LeVine, R. "A Cross-Cultural Perspective on Parenting." Pp. 17–26 in *Parenting in a Multicultural Society*, edited by M. Fantini and R. Cardenes. New York: Longman, 1980.

Lewando-Hundt, G., S. Beckerleg, F. Kassem, A.M.A. Jafar, I. Belmaker, K.A. Saad, and I. Shoham-Vardi. "Women's Health Custom Made: Building on the 40 Days Postpartum for Arab Women." *Health Care for Women International* 21 (2000): 529–542.

Li, R., and L. Grummer-Strawn. "Racial and Ehnic Disparities among United States Infants: Third National Health and Nutrition Survey, 1988–1994." *Birth* 29 (2002): 251–257.

Liam, I.I.L. "The Challenge of Migrant Motherhood: The Childrearing Practices of Chinese First-Time Mothers in Australia." Pp. 135–160 in *Asian Mothers, Western Birth*, edited by Pranee Liamputtong Rice. Melbourne: Ausmed Publications, 1999.

Liamputtong, P. "Motherhood and the Challenge of Immigrant Mothers: A Personal Reflection." *Families in Society* 82(2) (2001): 195–201.

Liamputtong, P. "Infant Feeding Practices: The Case of Hmong Women in Australia." *Health Care for Women International* 23(1) (2002): 33–48.

Liamputtong, P. "Motherhood and 'Moral Career': Discourses of Good Motherhood Among Southeast Asian Immigrant Women in Australia." *Qualitative Sociology* 29(1) (2006): 25–53.

Liamputtong P., and D. Ezzy. *Qualitative Research Methods*, 2nd edition. Melbourne: Oxford University Press, 2005.

Liamputtong, P., and C. Naksook. "Perceptions and Experiences of Motherhood, Health and the Husband's Roles among Thai Women in Australia." *Midwifery* 19(1) (2003a): 27–36.

Liamputtong, P., and C. Naksook. "Life as Mothers in a New Land: The Experience of Motherhood among Thai Women in Melbourne." *Health Care for Women International* 24(7) (2003b): 650–668.

Liamputtong, P., J.L. Halliday, R. Warren, L.F. Watson, and R.J. Bell. "Why Do Women Decline Prenatal Screening and Diagnosis: The Australian Womens Perspective." *Women & Health* 37 (2003): 89–108.

Liamputtong, P., S. Yimyam, S Parisunyakul, C. Baosoung, and N. Sansiriphun. "Women as Mothers: The Case of Thai Women in Northern Thailand." *International Social Work* 45(4) (2002): 497–515.

Liamputtong, P., S. Yimyam, S Parisunyakul, C. Baosoung, and N. Sansiriphun. "Pregnancy and Childbirth: Traditional Beliefs and Practices among Women in Chiang Mai, Northern Thailand." *Midwifery* 12(2) (2005): 139–153.

Liamputtong Rice, P. *Health and Sickness: The Influence of Cultural Knowledge and Commonsense Interpretations Among Thai Schoolchildren*. PhD thesis, Melbourne: Faculty of Education, Monash University, 1988.

Liamputtong Rice, P. "Infant Weaning Practices Among Hmong Women in Melbourne." *Australian Journal of Primary Health—Interchange* 5 (1999): 15–22.

Liamputtong Rice, P. *Hmong Women and Reproduction.* Westport, CT: Bergin & Garvey, 2000a.

Liamputtong Rice, P. "*Nyo Dua Hli*—30 Days Confinement: Traditions and Changed Childbearing Beliefs and Practices among Hmong Women in Australia." *Midwifery* 16 (2000b): 22–34.

Liamputtong Rice, P. "Baby, Souls, Name and Health: Traditional Customs for a Newborn Infant among the Hmong in Melbourne." *Early Human Development* 57 (2000c): 189–203.

Liamputtong Rice, P., and L. Manderson. (ed.) *Maternity and Reproductive Health in Asian Societies.* Amsterdam: Harwood Academic Press, 1996.

Liamputtong, P., and C. Naksook. "Caesarean or Vaginal Birth! Perceptions and Experience of Thai Mothers in Australian Hospitals." *Australian and New Zealand Journal of Public Health* 22 (1998a): 604–608.

Liamputtong, P., and C. Naksook. "The Experience of Pregnancy, Labour and Birth of Thai Women in Australia." *Midwifery* 14 (1998b): 74–84.

Liamputtong Rice, P., C. Naksook. "Breastfeeding Practices Among Thai Mothers in Melbourne." *Midwifery* 17(1) (2001): 11–23.

Liamputtong Rice, P., C. Naksook, and L.E. Watson. "The Experiences of Postpartum Hospital Stay and Returning Home Among Thai Mothers in Australia." *Midwifery* 15 (1999): 47–57.

Liesto, K., M. Rosenberg, and L. Walloe. "Breast-Feeding Practice in Norway 1860–1984." *Journal of Biosocial Sciences* 20 (1988): 45–58.

Lim, L.L. "The Feminization of Labour in the Asia-Pacific Rim Countries: From Contributing to Economic Dynamism to Bearing the Brunt of Structural Adjustment." Pp. 176–209 in *Human Resource in Development Along the Asia-Pacific Rim*, edited by Naohiro Ogawa and Gavin Jones. Singapore: Oxford University Press, 1993.

Limanonda, B. "Exploring Women's Status in Contemporary Thailand." Pp. 247–261 in *Women in Asia: Tradition, Modernity and Globalization*, edited by Louise Edwards and Mina Roses. Sydney: Allen & Unwin, 2000.

Lindenbaum, S., and M. Lock., eds. *Knowledge, Power, and Practice: The Anthropology of Medicine in Everyday Life.* Berkeley: University of California Press, 1993.

Lock, M., and N. Scheper-Hughes. "A Critical-Interpretive Approach in Medical Anthropology: Rituals and Routines of Discipline and Dissent." Pp. 47–73 in *Medical Anthropology: A Handbook of Theory and Method*, edited by Thomas Johnson and Carolyn Sargent. Westport, CT: Greenwood Press, 1990.

Luke, C. *Feminisms and the Pedagogies of Everyday Life.* New York: State University of New York, 1996.

Lupton, D. "Risk as Moral Danger: The Social and Political Functions of Risk Discourse in Public Health." *The International Journal of Health Services* 23 (1993): 425–435.

Lupton, D. *Medicine as Culture, Illness, Disease and the Body in Western Societies.* London: Sage Publications, 1995.

Lupton, D. *The Imperative of Health: Public Health and the Regulated Body*. London: Sage Publications, 1995.

Lupton, D. "Your Life in Their Hands: Trust in the Medical Encounter." Pp. 102–120 in *Health and the Sociology of Emotions*, edited by Veronica James and Jonathan Gabe. London: Blackwell Publishers, 1996.

Lupton, D. "Comsumerism, Reflexivity and the Medical Encounter." *Social Science & Medicine* 45 (1997): 373–381.

Lupton, D. "Foucault and the Medicalisation Critique." Pp. 94–110 in *Foucault, Health and Medicine*, edited by Alan Petersen and Robin Bunton. London: Routledge, 1997.

Lupton, D. *Risk*. London: Routledge, 1999.

Lupton, D. "'A Love/Hate Relationship': The Ideals and Experiences of First-Time Mothers." *Journal of Sociology* 36 (2000): 50–63.

Lupton, D., and J. Fenwick. "'They've Forgotten that I'm the Mum': Constructing and Practicing Motherhood in Special Care Nurseries." *Social Science & Medicine* 53 (2001): 1011–1021.

Lytleton, C. "Magic Lipstick and Verbal Caress: Doubling Standards in Isan Village." Pp. 165–187 in *Coming of Age in South and Southeast Asia: Youth, Courtship and Sexuality*, edited by Lenore Manderson and Pranee Liamputtong. Surrey: Curzon Press, 2002.

Lyttleton, C. *Endangered Relations: Negotiating Sex and AIDS in Thailand*. Amsterdam: Harwood Academic Press, 2000.

MacCormack, C. P., ed. *Ethnography of Fertility and Birth*. London: Academic Press, 1982.

Macintyre, M., and L. Dennerstein. *Shifting Latitudes, Changing Attitudes: Immigrant Women's Health Experiences, Attitudes, Knowledge and Beliefs*. Melbourne: Key Centre for Women's Health in Society, The University of Melbourne, 1995.

Malik, I.A., N. Bukhtiari, M-J.D. Good, M. Iqbal, S. Azim, M. Nawaz, L. Ashraf, R. Bhatty, and A. Ahmed. "Mothers' Fear of Child Death Due to Acute Diarrhoea: A Study in Urban and Rural Communities in Northern Punjab, Pakistan." *Social Science & Medicine* 35(8) (1992): 1043–1053.

Malin, M., E. Hemminki, O. Raikkonen, S. Sihvo, and M-L. Perala. "What Do Women Want? Women's Experiences of Infertility Treatment." *Social Science & Medicine* 53 (2001): 123–133.

Manderson, L. "Roasting, Smoking and Dieting in Response to Birth: Malay Confinement in Cross-Cultural Perspectives." *Social Science & Medicine* 15B (1981): 509–529.

Manderson, L. "Bottle Feeding and Ideology in Colonial Malaya: The Production of Change." *International Journal of Health Services* 12(4) (1982): 597–616.

Manderson, L. "To Nurse and to Nurture: Breastfeeding in Australian Society." Pp. 162–186 in *Breastfeeding, Child Health and Child Spacing*, edited by Valerie Hull and Mayling Simpson. London: Croom-Helm, 1985.

Mandl, P-E. "Rooming-In: History, Advantages, and Methods." Pp. 286–294 in *Programmes to Promote Breastfeeding*, edited by Dereck B. Jelliffe and E.F. Patrice Jelliffe. Oxford: Oxford University Press, 1988.

Manne, A. *Motherhood: How Should We Care for Our Children?* Sydney: Allen & Unwin, 2005.

Marchand, L., and M.H. Morrow. "Infant Feeding Practices: Understanding the Decision-Making Process." *Family Medicine* 26(5) (1994): 319–324.

Markens, S., C. H. Browner, and N. Press. "'Because of the Risks': How US Women Account for Refusing Prenatal Screening." *Social Science and Medicine* 49 (1999): 359–369.

Martin, E. "The Ideology of Reproduction: The Reproduction of Ideology." Pp. 300–314 in *Uncertain Terms: Negotiating Gender in American Society*, edited by Faye Ginsburg and Anna L. Tsing. Boston: Beacon Press, 1990.

Martin, E. *The Woman in the Body: A Cultural Analysis of Reproduction.* Boston: Beacon Press, 1992.

Mason, A., and B. Campbell. "Demographic Change and the Thai Economy: An Overview." Pp. 1–52 in *The Economic Impact of Demographic Change in Thailand, 1980–2015*, edited by B. Campbell, A. Mason, and E. Pernia. Honolulu: University of Hawaii Press, 1993.

Matich, J.R., and L.S. Sims. "A Comparison of Social Support Variables Between Women Who Intend to Breast or Bottle Feed." *Social Science & Medicine* 34 (1992): 919–927.

Maushart, S. *The Mask of Motherhood: How Mothering Changes Everything and Why We Pretend It Doesn't.* Sydney: Vintage, 1997.

Maxwell, N.E. "Modernization and Mobility into the Patrimonial Medical Elite in Thailand." *American Journal of Sociology* 810(3) (1975): 465–490.

Mayall, B., and M.C. Foster. *Child Health Care: Living with Children, Working for Children.* Oxford: Heineman Nursing, 1989.

McClain, C. "Ethno-Obstetrics in Ajijic." *Anthropology Quarterly* 48 (1975): 38–56.

McClain, C.S. "The Making of a Medical Tradition: Vaginal Birth after Cesarean." *Social Science & Medicine* 31(2) (1990): 203–210.

McHugh, P. "A Commonsense Conception of Deviance." Pp. 61–88 in *Deviance and Responsibility: The Social Construction of Moral Meanings*, edited by Jack D. Douglas. New York: Basic Books, 1970.

McKenna, J.J. "Cultural Influences on Infant and Childhood Sleep Biology, and the Science That Studies It: Toward a More Inclusive Paradigm." Pp. 199–230 in *Sleep and Breathing in Children: A Developmental Approach*, edited by Gerald M. Loughlin, John L. Carroll and Carole L. Marcus. New York: Marcel Dekker, 2000.

McMahon, M. *Engendering Motherhood: Identity and Self-Transformation in Women's Lives.* New York: The Guilford Press, 1995.

McNee, A., N. Khan, S. Dawson, J. Gunsalam, V. Tallo, L. Manderson, and I. Riley. "Responding to Cough: Boholano Illness Classification and Resort to Care in Response to Childhood ARI." *Social Science & Medicine* 40(9) (1995): 1279–1289.

Mechanic, D. "Public Trust and Initiatives for New Health Care Partnerships." *The Millbank Quarterly* 76 (1998): 281–302.

Mechanic, D., and S. Meyer. "Concepts of Trust among Patients with Serious Illness." *Social Science & Medicine* 51(5) (2000): 657–668.

Millard, A.V. "The Place of the Clock in Pediatric Advice: Rationales, Cultural Themes, and Impediments to Breastfeeding." *Social Science & Medicine* 31 (1990): 211–221.

Milligan, R.A., L.C. Pugh, and Y.L. Bronner. "Breastfeeding Duration among Low Income Women." *Journal of Midwifery and Women's Health* 45(3) (2000): 246–252.

Mills, M.B. *Thai Women in the Global Labor Force: Consuming Desires, Contested Selves*. New Brunswick: Rutgers University Press, 1999.

Ministry of Public Health. *Thailand: Basic Health, Population & Reproductive Health Information*. Bangkok: Ministry of Public Health, 2002.

Ministry of Public Health Thailand: Country' Health Profile, 2002. http://eng.moph .go.th/profile97–98/content.tem.

Misztal, B. *Trust in Modern Societies: The Search for the Bases of Social Order*. Cambridge: Polity Press, 1996.

Moffat, T. "Breastfeeding, Wage Labour, and Insufficient Milk in Peri-Urban Kathmandu, Nepal." *Medical Anthropology* 21 (2002): 165–188.

Moon Park, E., and G. Dimigen. "Cross-Cultural Comparison of the Social Support System after Childbirth." *Journal of Comparative Family Studies* 25(3) (1994): 3–10.

Mooney, G.H., and M. Ryan. "Agency in Health Care: Getting Beyond First Principles." *Journal of Health Economics* 12 (1993): 125–135.

Morelli, G.A., D. Oppenheim, B. Rogoff, and D. Goldsmith, D. "Cultural Variation in Infants' Sleeping Arrangements: Questions of Independence." *Developmental Psychology* 28(4) (1992): 604–613.

Morrison, L. "Traditions in Transition: Young People's Risk for HIV in Chiang Mai, Thailand." *Qualitative Health Research* 14(3) (2004): 328–344.

Morse, J.M. "The Cultural Context of Infant Feeding in Fiji." *Ecology of Food and Nutrition* 14 (1984): 287–296.

Morse, J.M. "The Cultural Context of Infant Feeding in Fiji." Pp. 255–268 in *Infant Care and Feeding in the South Pacific*, edited by Leslie B. Marshall. New York: Gordon and Breach, 1985.

Morse, J.M., C. Jehle, and D. Gamble. "Initiating Breastfeeding: A World Survey of the Timing of Postpartum Breastfeeding." *International Journal of Nursing Studies* 3 (1990): 303–313.

Morse, J.M., J.L. Bottorff, and J. Boman. "Patterns of Breastfeeding and Work: The Canadian Experience." *Canadian Journal of Public Health* 80(3) (1989): 182–188.

Moss, P., G. Bolland, R. Foxman, and C. Owen. "The Hospital Inpatient Stay: The Experience of First-Time Parents." *Child: Care, Health and Development* 13 (1987): 153–167.

Mougne, C. "An Ethnography of Reproduction: Changing Patterns of Fertility in a Northern Thai Village." Pp. 68–106 in *Nature and Man in South East Asia*, edited by Philip A. Stott. London: School of Oriental and African Studies, University of London, 1978.

Moustakas, C. *Phenomenological Research Methods*. Thousand Oaks: Sage, 1994.

Muecke, M. "Health Care Systems as Socializing Agents: Childbearing the North Thai and Western Ways." *Social Science & Medicine* 10 (1976): 337–383.

Muecke, M. "Make Money Not Babies: Changing Status Markers of Northern Thai Women." *Asian Survey* 24(4) (1984): 459–470.

Mulder, N. *Everyday Life in Thailand: An Interpretation.* Bangkok: Duang Kamol, 1985.

Murphy, E. "'Breast is Best': Infant Feeding Decisions and Maternal Deviance." *Sociology of Health & Illness* 21 (1999): 187–208.

Murphy, E. "Risk, Responsibility, and Rhetoric in Infant Feeding." *Journal of Contemporary Ethnography* 29(3) (2000): 291–325.

Murray, S.F. "Relation between Private Health Insurance and High Rates of Caesarean Section in Chile: Qualitative and Quantitative Study." *British Medical Journal* 321 (2000): 1501–1505.

Nadesan, M.H., and P. Sotirin. "The Romance and Science of 'Breast is Best': Discursive Contradictions and Contexts of Breast-Feeding Choices." *Text and Performance Quarterly* 18 (1998): 217–232.

Naksook, C., and P. Liamputtong Rice. "'Can He Be Born on Tuesday, Doctor?' Traditional and Changed Beliefs and Practices Related to Birth Among Thai Women in Australia." Pp. 237–252 in *Asian Mothers, Western Birth*, edited by Pranee Liamputtong Rice. Melbourne: Ausmed Publications, 1999.

Nardi, B.A. "Infant Feeding and Women's Work in Western Samoa: A Hypothesis, Some Evidence and Suggestions." Pp. 293–306 in *Infant Care and Feeding in the South Pacific*, edited by Leslie B. Marshall. Gordon and Breach, New York, 1985.

National Center for Health Statistics. *Healthy People 2000 Review, 1995–96.* DHHS (PHS) Publication No. 96–1256. Hyattsville, MD: National Center for Health Statistics, 1996.

National Economic and Development Board (NESDB). *Thailand: National Report on Population and Development.* A report prepared by Thailand Working Committee for preparation of the International Conference on Population and Development (September). Bangkok: NESDB, 1994.

National Economic and Social Development Board. *The Seventh National Economic and Social Development Plan (1992–1996).* Bangkok: National Economic and Social Development Board, Office of the Prime Minister, 1992.

National Statistical Office. *The 1996 Survey of Fertility in Thailand.* Bangkok: National Statistical Office, 1997.

Nations, M.K., and L.A. Rebhun. "Angels with Wet Wings Won't Fly: Maternal Sentiment in Brazil and the Image of Neglect." *Culture, Medicine & Psychiatry* 12 (1988): 141–200.

Nelson, M.K. "Working-Class Women, Middle-Class Women, and Models of Childbirth." *Social Problems* 30(3) (1983): 284–297.

Newman, J. "How Breast Milk Protects Newborns." *Scientific American* 4 (1995): 76–79.

Nichter, M., and M. Nichter. "The Ethnophysiology and Folk Dietetics of Pregnancy: A Case Study from South India." Pp. 35–69 in *Anthropology and International Health: Asian Case Studies*, edited by Mark Nichter and Mimi Nichter. Amsterdam: Gordon and Breach Publishers, 1996.

Novas, C., and N. Rose. "Genetic Risk and the Birth of the Somatic Individual." *Economy & Society* 29(4) (2000): 485–513.

Oakley, A. *Becoming a Mother*. Oxford: Martin Roberson, 1979.

Oakley, A. *Women Confined: Towards a Sociology of Childbirth*. Oxford: Martin Robertson, 1980.

Oakley, A. *The Captured Womb: A History of the Medical Care in Pregnant Women*. New York: Basel Blackwell, 1986.

Oakley, A. "Is Social Support Good for the Health of Mothers and Babies?" *Journal of Reproductive & Infant Psychology* 6 (1988): 3–21.

Oakley, A. *Responding to the Health Needs of Women in Pregnancy and the First Year of Motherhood. Social Support and Maternity and Child Health Services: A Guide to Good Practice for NHS Purchasers*. Salford: Public Health Research and Resource Centre, 1993.

Oakley, A., and L. Rajan. "Social Class and Social Support: The Same or Different?" *Sociology* 25 (1991): 31–59.

Oakley, A., L. Rajan, and A. Grant. "Social Support and Pregnancy Outcome." *British Journal of Obstetrics and Gynaecology* 97 (1990): 155–162.

O'Barr, J., Pope, D., and M. Wher. Pp. 1–14 in Introduction to *Ties that Bind: Essays on Mothering and Patriarchy*, edited by Jean O'Barr, Deborah Pope and Mary Wyer. Chicago: University of Chicago Press, 1990.

O'Gara, C. "Breastfeeding and Maternal Employment in Urban Honduras." Pp. 113–130 in *Women, Work and Child Welfare in the Third World*, edited by Joanne Leslie and Michael Paolisso. Boulder, Colorado: Westview Press, 1989.

Olin Lauritzen, S. "Notions of Child Health: Mothers' Accounts of Health in Their Young Babies." *Sociology of Health & Illness* 19(4) (1997): 436–456.

Olin Lauritzen, S., and L. Sachs. "Normality, Risk and the Future: Implicit Communication of Threat in Health Surveillance." *Sociology of Health & Illness* 23 (2001): 497–516.

Ortner, S. "Is Female to Male as Nature is to Culture?" Pp. 67–87 in *Women, Culture and Society*, edited by Michelle Zimbalist Rosaldo and Louise Lamphere. Stanford: Stanford University Press, 1974.

Osborne, T. "Of Health and Statecraft." Pp. 173–188 in *Foucault, Health and Medicine*, edited by Alan Petersen and Robin Bunton. London: Routledge, 1997.

Parson, T. *The Social System*. Glencoe, Ill: Free Press, 1951.

Philipona, J. "L'Allaitement Maternel en Europe." *Les dossiers de l'obstetrique* 216 (1994): 38–40.

Phillips, D. "Medical Professional Dominance and Client Dissatisfaction: A Study of Doctor-Patient Interaction and Reported Dissatisfaction with Medical Care among Female Patients at Four Hospitals in Trinidad and Tobago." *Social Science & Medicine* 42 (1996): 1419–1425.

Phillips, H.P. *Thai Peasant Personality*. Berkeley: University of California Press, 1965.

Phoenix, A., and A. Woollett. "Motherhood: Social Construction, Politics and Psychology." Pp. 13–27 in *Motherhood: Meanings, Practices and Ideologies*, edited by Ann Phoenix, Anne Woollett, and Eva Lloyd. London: Sage Publications, 1991.

Pillsbury, B.L.K. "'Doing the Month': Confinement and Convalescence of Chinese Women after Childbirth." *Social Science & Medicine* 12 (1978): 11–22.

Podhisita, C. "Buddhism and Thai World View." In *Traditional and Changing Thai World View*, edited by Chulalongkorn University Social Research Institute. Bangkok: Chulalongkorn University, 1985.

Podhisita, C., N. Havanon, J. Knodel, and W. Sittitrai. "Women's Work and Family Size in Rural Thailand." *Asia-Pacific Population Journal* 5(2) (1990): 31–52.

Porter, M., and S. Macintyre. "What Is, Must Be Best: A Research Note on Conservative or Deferential Responses to Antenatal Care Provision." *Social Science & Medicine* 19(11) (1984): 1197–1200.

Potter, J.E., E. Berquo, I.H.O. Perpe, O.F. Leal, K. Hopkins, M.R. Sou, and M.C. Formiga. "Unwanted Caesarean Sections among Public and Private Patients in Brazil: Prospective Study." *British Medical Journal* 323(7322) (2001): 1155–1159.

Potter, S.H. *Family Life in a Northern Thai Village: A Study in the Structural Significance of Women.* Berkeley: University of California Press, 1977.

Poulsen, A. *Pregnancy and Childbirth—Its Customs and Rites in a North-Eastern Thai Village.* Copenhagen: Danish International Development Agency, 1983.

Pramualratana, A. "The Impact of Societal Change and Role of the Old in a Rural Community in Thailand." Pp. 44–54 in *Changing Roles and Statuses of Women in Thailand*, edited by Bencha Yoddumnern-Attig. Salaya: Institute for Population and Social Research, Mahidol University, 1992.

Pyne, H.H. "Reproductive Experiences and Needs of Thai Women: Where Has Development Taken Us?" Pp. 19–41 in *Power and Decision: The Social Control of Reproduction*, edited by G. Sen and R.C. Snow. Harvard University Press, 1994.

Quarles, A., P.D. William, D.A. Hoyle, M. Brimeyer, and A.R. William. "Mother's Intention, Age, Education and Duration and Management of Breastfeeding." *Maternal-Child Nursing Journal* 22(3) (1994): 102–107.

Quine, L., D.R. Rutter, and S. Gowen. "Women's Satisfaction with the Quality of the Birth Experience: A Prospective Study of Social and Psychological Predictors." *Journal of Reproductive and Infant Psychology* 11 (1993): 107–113.

Ram, K. "Medical Management and Giving Birth: Responses of Coastal Women in Tamil Nadu." *Reproductive Health Matters* 4 (1994): 20–26.

Raphael, D. *Being Female: Reproduction, Power, and Change.* Mouton Press: The Hague, 1975.

Rapp, R. "Moral Pioneers: Women, Men, and Fetuses on a Frontier of Reproductive Technology." Women & Health 13(1–2) (1987): 101–116.

Rapp, R. "Accounting for Amniocentesis." Pp. 55–76 in *Knowledge, Power, and Practice: The Anthropology of Medicine in Everyday Life*, edited by Shirley Lindenbaum and Magaret Lock. Berkeley: University of California Press, 1993.

Rapp, R. "Risky Business: Genetic Counselling in a Shifting World." Pp. 175-189 in *Articulating hidden histories*, edited by Jane Schneider and Rayna Rapp. Berkeley: University of California Press, 1995.

Rapp, R. "Refusing Prenatal Diagnosis: The Meanings of Bioscience in a Multicultural World." Science, *Technology, and Human Values* 23 (1998): 45–70.

Rapp, R. *Testing Women, Testing the Fetus: The Social Impact of Amniocentesis in America*. New York: Routledge, 1999.

Rasmussen, N., and P. Moss, eds. *L'Emploi Des Parents et la Garde des Enfants*. Le Ministere des Afaires Sociales, Copenhague, 1993.

Reichart, J.A., M. Baron., and J. Fawcett. "Changes in Attitudes toward Caesarean Birth." *Journal of Obstetric, Gynecologic & Neonatal Nursing* 22(2) (1993): 159–167.

Rendina, T., and P. Liamputtong. "Prenatal Expectations: The Effects on the Experiences of Motherhood and the Mothering Role Among Australian women." Unpublished paper submitted for publication, 2006.

Rhodes, L. "Studying Biomedicine as a Cultural System." Pp. 159–174 in *Medical Anthropology: A Handbook of Theory and Method*, edited by Thomas Johnson and Carolyn Sargent. Westport, CT: Greenwood Press, 1990.

Rhum, M. *Ancestral Lords: Gender, Dissent and Spirits in a Northern Thai Village*. Dekalb: Northern Illinois University, Center for Southeast Asian Studies, 1994.

Ribbens, J., J. McCarthy, R. Edwards, and V. Gllies. "Moral Tales of the Child and the Adult: Narratives of Contemporary Family Lives under Changing Circumstances." *Sociology* 34(4) (2000): 785–803.

Ribbens, J. *Mothers and Their Children: A Feminist Sociology of Childrearing*. London: Sage Publications, 1994.

Rice, P.L. "Culture and Infant Feeding Practices among Southeast Asian Mothers Living in Melbourne." *Birth Issues* 7(1) (1998): 15–22.

Rice, P.L., and C. Naksook. "Childrearing and Cultural Beliefs and Practices among Thai Mothers in Victoria: Implications for the Sudden Infant Death Syndrome." *Journal of Peadiatrics & Child Health* 34(4) (1998): 302–306.

Rice, P. L. "What Women Say about Their Childbirth Experiences: The Case of Hmong Women in Australia." *Journal of Reproductive & Infant Psychology* 17(3) (1999a): 237–253.

Rice, P. L. "Rooming-In and Cultural Practices: Choice or Constraint?" *Journal of Reproductive & Infant Psychology* 18(1) (1999b): 21–32.

Richardson, D. *Women, Motherhood and Children*. London: Macmillan, 1993.

Richter, K., and B. Yoddumnern-Attig. "Framing a Study of Thai Women's Changing Roles and Statuses." Pp. 1–7 in *Changing Roles and Statuses of Women in Thailand: A Documentary Assessment*, edited by Bencha Yoddumnern-Attig, Kerry Richter, Amara Soonthorndhada, Chanya Sethaput, and Anthony Pramualratana. Salaya: The Institute for Population and Social Research, Mahidol University, 1992.

Riewpaiboon, W., K. Chuengsatiansup, L. Gilson, and V. Tangcharoensathien. "Private Obstetric Practice in a Public Hospital: Mythical Trust in Obstetric Care." *Social Science & Medicine* 61 (2005): 1408–1417.

Riley, J.N. "Western Medicine's Attempt to Become More Scientific: Examples from the United States and Thailand." *Social Science & Medicine* 11(10) (1977): 549–560.

Riordan, J. "Cost of Not Breastfeeding: A Commentary." *Journal of Human Lactation* 13 (1997): 93–97.

Robinson, J.B., A.E. Hunt, J. Pope, and B. Garner. "Attitudes toward Infant Feeing Among Adolescent Mothers from a WIC Population in Northern Louisiana." *Journal of American Diet Association* 93 (1993): 1311–1313.

Romalis, S. *Childbirth: Alternatives to Medical Control.* Austin: University of Texas Press, 1981.

Romito, P., and M-J. Saurel-Cubizolles. "Working Women and Breast-Feeding: The Experience of First-Time Mothers in an Italian Town." *Journal of Reproductive & Infant Psychology* 14 (1996): 145–156.

Root, R, and C. Browner. "Practices of the Pregnant Self: Compliance With and Resistance to Prenatal Norms." *Culture, Medicine & Psychiatry* 25 (2001): 195–223.

Ross Laboratories. *Ross Laboratories Mothers' Survey: 1986–1994.* Unpublished report, Ross Laboratories, Columbus, OH, 1995.

Rossiter, J.C. "Maternal-Infant Health Beliefs and Infant Feeding Practices: The Perception and Experience of Immigrant Vietnamese Women." Pp. 161–174 in *Asian Mothers, Australian Birth. Pregnancy, Childbirth and Childrearing: The Asian Experience in an English-Speaking Country*, edited by Pranee Liamputtong Rice. Melbourne: Ausmed Publications, 1994.

Rossiter, J.C. "Attitudes of Vietnamese Women to Baby Feeding Practices Before and After Immigration to Sydney." *Midwifery* 8 (1992): 103–112.

Rothman, B.K. *Recreating Motherhood: Ideology and Technology in a Patriarchal Society.* New York: W.W. Norton, 1989.

Ruddick, S. "Maternal Thinking." *Feminist Studies* 6 (1980): 342–364.

Ryan, A.S., and G.A. Martinez. "Breast-Feeding and the Working Mothers: A Profile." *Pediatrics* 83(4) (1989): 524–531.

Ryan, A.S., D. Rush, F.W. Krieger, and G.E. Lewandowski. "Recent Declines in Breastfeeding in the United States, 1984–1989." *Pediatrics* 88 (1991): 719–727.

Sabo, D., and D.F. Gordon. *Men's Health and Illness: Gender, Power and the Body.* Thousand Oaks: Sage Publications, 1995.

Sakala, C. "Medically Unnecessary Caesarean Section Births: Introduction to a Symposium." *Social Science & Medicine* 37 (1993): 1177–1198.

Salmon, P., and N.C. Drew. "Multidimentional Assessment of Women's Experience of Childbirth: Relationship to Obstetric Procedure, Antenatal Preparation and Obstetric History." *Journal of Psychosomal Research* 36 (1992): 317–327.

Sargent, C. "Solitary Confinement: Birth Practices Among the Bariba of the People's Republic of Benin." Pp. 193-210 in *Anthropology of Human Birth*, edited by Margarita Kay. Philadelphia: F. A. Davis Company, 1982.

Sargent, C., and G. Bascope. "Ways of Knowing about Birth in Three Cultures." *Medical Anthropology Quarterly* 10(2) (1996): 213–236.

Sawicki, J. *Disciplining Foucault: Feminism, Power, and the Body.* New York: Routledge, 1991.

Scheper-Hughes, N. "Infant Mortality and Infant Care: Cultural and Economic Constraints on Nurturing in Northeast Brazil." *Social Science & Medicine* 19(5) (1984): 535–546.

Scheper-Hughes, N. "Culture, Scarcity, and Maternal Thinking: Maternal Detachment and Infant Survival in Brazilian Shantytown." *Ethos* 13 (1985): 291–317.

Scheper-Hughes, N. "Culture, Scarcity, and Maternal Thinking: Mother Love and Child Death in Northeast Brazil." Pp. 187–208 in *Child Survival: Anthropological Perspectives on the Treatment and Maltreatment of Children*, edited by Nancy Scheper-Hughes. Dordrecht: D. Reidel Publishing Company, 1987a.

Scheper-Hughes, N. "The Cultural Politics of Child Survival." Pp. 1–29 in *Child Survival: Anthropological Perspectives on the Treatment and Maltreatment of Children*, edited by Nancy Scheper-Hughes. Dordrecht: D. Reidel Publishing Company, 1987b.

Scheper-Hughes, N. "The Madness of Hunger: Sickness, Delirium, and Human Needs." *Culture, Medicine & Psychiatry* 12 (1988): 429–458.

Scheper-Hughes, N. "Social Indifference to Child Death." *Lancet* 337 (1991): 1144–1147.

Scheper-Hughes, N. *Death Without Weeping: The Violence of Everyday Life in Brazil.* Berkeley: University of California Press, 1992.

Schmied, V., and D. Lupton. "Blurring the Boundaries: Breastfeeding and Maternal Subjectivity." *Sociology of Health & Illness* 23(2) (2001): 234–250.

Scott, J.A., and C.W. Binns. "Factors Associated with the Initiation and Duration of Breastfeeding: A Review of Literature." *Breastfeeding Reviews* 7 (1999): 5–16.

Scott, M.B., and S.M. Lyman. "Accounts." *American Sociological Review* 33 (1963): 46–62.

Scott, S., L. Prior, F. Wood, and J. Gray. "Repositioning the Patient: The Implications of Being 'At Risk.'" *Social Science & Medicine* 60 (2005): 1869–1879.

Selvaratnam, S. "Population and Status of Women." *Asia-Pacific Population Journal* 3(2) (1988): 3–23.

Sermsri, S. "Utilization of Traditional and Modern Health Care Services in Thailand." Pp. 160–179 in *The Triumph of Practicality: Tradition and Modernity in Health Care Utilization in Selected Asian Countries*, edited by Stella R. Quah. Singapore: Institute of Southeast Asian Studies, 1989.

Sharpe, Sue. *Double Identity: The Lives of Working Mothers.* Harmondsworth: Penguin Books, 1984.

Sheehan, A. *Complex Decisions: Deconstructing Best—A Grounded Theory Study of Infant Feeding Decisions in the First Six Weeks Post Birth.* Unpublished doctoral thesis, University of Technology, Sydney, 2006.

Shildrick, M. *Leaky Bodies and Boundaries: Feminism, Postmodernism and (Bio) Ethics.* London: Routledge, 1997.

Sich, D. "Traditional Concepts and Customs on Pregnancy, Birth and Post Partum Period in Rural Korea." *Social Science and Medicine* 15B (1981): 65-69.

Simons, W. "Watching the Clock: Keeping Time during Pregnancy, Birth and Postpartum Experiences." *Social Science & Medicine* 55 (2002): 559–570.

Sitthi-amorn, C., R. Somrongthong, and W.S. Janjaroen. "Globalization and Health Viewed from Three Parts of the World." *Bulletin of the World Health Organization* 79 (2001): 889–894.

Small, R., P. Liamputtong Rice, J. Yelland, and J. Lumley. "Mothers in a New Country: The Role of Culture and Communication in Vietnamese, Turkish and Filipino

Women's Experiences of Giving Birth in Australia." *Women & Health* 22(3) (1999): 77–101.

Small, R., J. Yelland, J. Lumley, S. Brown, and P. Liamputtong. "Immigrant Women's Views about Care During Labor and Birth: An Australian Study of Vietnamese, Turkish and Filipino Women." *Birth* 29(4) (2002): 266–277.

Smart, C. "Disruptive Bodies and Unruly Sex." Pp. 5–32 in *Regulating Womanhood: Historical Essays on Marriage, Motherhood and Sexuality*, edited by C. Smart. New York: Routledge, 1992.

Smith, T.E. *The Politic of Family Planning in the Third World*. London: Allen & Unwin, 1973.

Snow, L.F., and S.M. Johnson. "Folklore, Food, Female Reproductive Cycle." *Ecology of Food & Nutrition* 7 (1978): 41–49.

Spisak, S., and S.S. Gross. *Second Follow-up Report: The Surgeon General's Workshop on Breastfeeding and Human Lactation*. Washington, D.C.: National Center for Education in Maternal and Child Health, 1991.

Squire, C. *Significant Differences: Feminism in Psychology*. London: Sage, 1989.

Stallybrass, P., and A. White. *The Politics and Poetics of Transgression*. Ithaca: Cornell University Press, 1989.

Stanway, P., and A. Stanway. *Breast is Best: A Commonsense Approach to Breast Feeding*. London: Pan Books, 1978.

Stein, H. *American Medicine as Culture*. Boulder, CO: Westview Press, 1990.

Steinberg, S. "Childbearing Research: A Transcultural Review." *Social Science & Medicine* 43(2) (1996): 1765–1784.

Straten, G.F.M., R.D. Friele, and P.P. Groenewegen. "Public Trust in Dutch Health Care." *Social Science & Medicine* 55 (2002): 227–234.

Strauss, A.L. *Qualitative Analysis for Social Scientists*. Cambridge: Cambridge University Press, 1987.

Surasiengsunk, S., S. Kiranandana, K. Wongboonsin, G. Garnett, R. Anderson, and G. van Griensven. "Demographic Impact of the HIV Epidemic in Thailand." *AIDS* 12 (1998): 775–784.

Suvanajata, T. "Is Thai Social System Loosely Structured?" *Journal of Social Science Review* 1(1976): 171–188.

Sykes, D.M., and D. Matza. "Techniques of Neutralization: A Theory of Delinquency." *American Sociological Review* 22(6) (1957): 664–670.

Symonds, P.V. *Cosmology and the Cycle of Life: Hmong Views of Birth, Death and Gender in a Mountain Village in Northern Thailand*. Rhode Island: Brown University, 1991.

Symonds, P.V. "Journey to the Land of Light: Birth Among Hmong Women." Pp. 103–123 in *Maternity and Reproductive Health in Asian Societies*, edited by Pranee Liamputtong Rice and Lenore Manderson. Amsterdam: Harwood Academic Publishers, 1996.

Szasz, T.S., and M.H. Hollenger. "A Contribution to the Philosophy of Medicine: The Basic Models of the Doctor-Patient Relationship." *American Medical Association Archives of Internal Medicine* 97 (1956): 585–592.

Takrudtong, M. "Reproductive Health in Thailand: Issues of Interest. Fact sheet—Family Planning and Population." 1(11) (August, 1–4, 1998). http://www.anamai .moph.go.th/factsheet/health1–11_en.htm.

Tantiwiramanond, D., and R.S. Pandey. "Status and Role of Thai Women in the Pre-Modern Period: A Historical and Cultural Perspective." *Sojourn* 2(1) (1987): 125–149.

Tantiwiramanond, D., and R.S. Pandey. "New Opportunities or New Inequalities: Development Issues and Women's Lives in Thailand." Pp. 83–135 in *Women, Gender Relations and Development in Thai Society*, edited by Virada Somswasdi and Sally Theobald. Chiang Mai: Women Studies Centre, Faculty of Social Sciences, Chiang Mai University, 1997.

Tantiwiramanond, D., and R.S. Pandey. *By Women, For Women: A Study of Women's Organizations in Thailand*. Pasir Panjang Singapore: Institute of Southeast Asian Studies, 1991.

Tarkka, M., and M. Paunonen. "Social Support and Its Impact on Mother's Experiences of Childbirth." *Journal of Advanced Nursing* 23 (1996): 70–75.

Tatar, M., S. Gunalp, S. Somunoglu, and A. Demirol. "Women's Perceptions of Caesarean Section: Reflections from a Turkish Teaching Hospital." *Social Science & Medicine* 50 (2000): 1227–1233.

Thailand Country Health Profile (2004). Internet access: http://w3.whosea.org/cntry-health/thailand/women.html (accessed May 21, 2004).

Thitsa, K. *Providence and Prostitution: Women in Buddhist Thailand*. London: Change International Reports, 1980.

Thoits, P.A. "Conceptual, Methodological, and Theoretical Problems in Studying Social Support as a Buffer Against Life Stress." *Journal of Health & Social Behaviour* 23 (1982): 145–159.

Thoits, P.A. "Social Support as Coping Assistance." *Journal of Consulting & Clinical Psychology* 54 (1986): 416–423.

Thurer, S.L. *The Myths of Motherhood: How Culture Reinvents the Good Mother*. Boston: Houghton Mifflin Company, 1994.

Timbo, B., S. Altekruse, M. Headrick, and K. Klontz. Breastfeeding among Black Mothers: Evidence Supporting the Need for Prenatal Intervention. *Journal of Social Pediatrics and Nursing* 1(1) (1996): 35–40.

Townsend, K., and P. Liamputtong Rice. "A Baby Is Born in Site 2 Camp: Pregnancy, Birth and Confinement among Cambodian Refugee Women." Pp. 125–143 in *Maternity and Reproductive Health in Asian Societies*, edited by Pranee Liamputtong Rice and Lenore Manderson. Amsterdam: Harwood Academic Publishers, 1996.

Tully, J., and K.G. Dewey. "Private Fears, Global Loss: A Cross-Cultural Study of the Insufficient Syndrome." *Medical Anthropology* 9 (1985): 225–243.

Turner, B.S. *Medical Power and Social Knowledge*, revised edition. London: Sage, 1995.

Turner, B.S. "From Governmentality to Risk: Some Reflections on Foucault's Contribution to Medical Sociology." Pp. viii–xxi in *Foucault, Health and Medicine*, edited by Alan Petersen and Robin Bunton. London: Routledge, 1997.

Turner, V. *The Forest of Symbols*. Ithaca: Cornell University Press, 1967.

Turner, V. "Betwixt and Between: The Liminal Period in Rites de Passage." Pp. 234–43 in *Reader in Comparative Religion*, edited by William Lessa and Evon Z. Vogt. . . . New York: Harper and Row, 1979.

UNICEF. Thailand, 2002. http://www.unicef.org/statis/country_1page174.html.

Ussher, J. "Negative Images of Female Sexuality and Reproduction: Reflecting Misogyny or Misinformation?" *Psychology of Women Newsletter* 5 (1990): 17–29.

Van Esterik, P. "Laywomen in Theravada Buddhism." Pp. 55–78 in *Women of Southeast Asia*, edited by Penny van Esterik. Wyoming: Northern Illinois University Press, 1982.

Van Esterik, P. "The Cultural Context of Breastfeeding in Rural Thailand." Pp. 139–161 in *Breastfeeding, Child Health and Child Spacing*, edited by Valerie Hull and Mayling Simpson. Croom Helm, London, 1985.

Van Esterik, P. "The Cultural Context of Infant Feeding." Pp. 187–201 in *Feeding Infants in Four Societies: Causes and Consequences of Mothers' Choices*, edited by Beverly Winikoff, Mary A. Castle and Virginia H. Laukaran. Greenwood Press, New York, 1988.

Van Esterik, P. *Beyond the Breast-Bottle Controversy*. Rutgers University Press, New Jersey, 1989.

Van Esterik, P., and M.A. Castle. "The Influence of Health Services." Pp. 121–146 in *Feeding Infants in Four Societies: Causes and Consequences of Mothers' Choices*, edited by B. Winikoff, M.A. Castle, and V.H. Laukaran. Greenwood Press, New York, 1988.

Van Esterik, P., and T. Greiner. "Breastfeeding and Women's Work: Constraints and Opportunities." *Studies in Family Planning* 12(4) (1981): 184–197.

Van Esterik, P., and L. Menon. *Being Mother-Friendly: A Practical Guide for Working Women and Breastfeeding*. Penang: World Alliance for Breastfeeding Action, 1996.

Van Gennep, A. *The Rites of Passage*. Chicago: University of Chicago Press, 1966.

Vichi-Vadakan, J. "Women and the Family in Thailand in the Midst of Social Change." *Law and Society Review* 28 (1994): 515–525.

Vincent, C., S.J. Ball, and S. Pietikainen. "Metropolitan Mothers: Mothers, Mothering and Paid Work." *Women's Studies International Forum* 27 (2004): 571–587.

Vong-Ek, P. "How Popular Beliefs Influence Breastfeeding Practices in Northeast and Central Thailand." *Journal of Primary Health Care & Development* 6 (1993): 61–76.

Wales, H.G.Q. *Divination in Thailand*. London: Curzon Press, 1983.

Walker, A. "A Fresh Look at the Risks of Artificial Infant Feeding." *Journal of Human Lactation* 9 (1993): 97–107.

Wantana, S. *Development of the Thai Working Class*. Bangkok: Thai Khadi Research Institute, Thammasat University, 1982.

Warakamin, S, and M. Takrudtong. "Reproductive Health in Thailand: An Overview. Fact Sheet, Family Planning and Population." 1(6) (March, 1–4, 1998). http://www.anamai.moph.go.th/factsheet/health1–6_en.htm.

Wearing, B. *The Ideology of Motherhood*. Sydney: George Allen & Unwin, 1984.

Weaver, J.J., and J.M. Ussher. "How Motherhood Changes Life: A Discourse Analytic Study with Mothers of Young Children." *Journal of Reproductive & Infant Psychology* 15 (1997): 51–68.

Weise, H.J.C. "Maternal Nutrition and Traditional Food Behavior in Haiti." *Human Organization* 35 (1976): 193–200.

Weller, S.C., and C.I. Dungy. "Personal Preferences and Ethnic Variations among Anglo and Hispanic Breast and Bottle Feeders." *Social Science & Medicine* 23 (1986): 539–548.

Wertz, R.W., and D.C. Wertz. *Lying-In: A History of Childbirth in America*. New York: Free Press, 1977.

Whelan, A., and P. Lupton. "Promoting Successful Breastfeeding among Women With a Low Income." *Midwifery* 14 (1998): 94–100.

White, A., S. Freeth, and M. O'Brien. *Infant Feeding 1990*. London: HMSO, 1992.

Whittaker, A. *Issan Women: Ethnicity, Gender and Health in Northeast Thailand*. PhD thesis, Brisbane: Tropical Health Program, The University of Queensland, 1995.

Whittaker, A. "Birthing, the Postpartum and Development: Ideology and Practice in Northeast Thailand." Pp. 469–498 in *Women, Gender Relations and Development in Thai Society*, edited by Virada Somswasdi and Sally Theobald. Chiang Mai: Chiang Mai University, 1997.

Whittaker, A. "Birth and the Postpartum in Northeast Thailand: Contesting Modernity and Tradition." *Medical Anthropology* 18 (1999): 215–242.

Whittaker, A. *Intimate Knowledge: Women and Their Health in North-East Thailand*. Sydney: Allen & Unwin, 2000.

Whittaker, A. "Water Serpents and Staying by the Fire: Markers of Maturity in a Northeast Thai Village." Pp. 17–41 in *Coming of Age in South and Southeast Asia: Youth, Courtship and Sexuality*, edited by Lenore Manderson and Pranee Liamputtong. Surrey: Curzon Press, 2002.

Wiemann, C.M., J.C. DuBois, and A.B. Berenson. "Racial/Ethnic Difference in the Decision to Breastfeed among Adolescent Mothers." *Pediatrics* 101 (1998): E11.

Wiles, R., and J. Higgins. "Doctor-Patient Relationship in the Private Sector: Patients' Perceptions." *Sociology of Health & Illness* 18 (1996): 341–356.

Williams, S.J. "Theorising Class, Health and Lifestyles: Can Bourdieu Help Us?" *Sociology of Health & Illness* 17(5) (1995): 577–604.

Wilmoth, T.A., and J.P. Elder. "An Assessment of Research on Breastfeeding Promotion Strategies in Developing Countries." *Social Science & Medicine* 41 (1995): 579–594.

Wilson, C.S. "Food Taboos of Childbirth: The Malay Example." *Ecology of Food & Nutrition* 2 (1973): 267–274.

Winichagoon, P., T. Viriyapanich, and S. Dhamamitta. "Breastfeeding in Thailand: Trends and Promotion Efforts." Pp. 124–132 in *Integrating Food and Nutrition into Development: Thailand's Experiences and Future Visions*, edited by P. Winichagoodm Y. Kachondham, G.A. Attig, and K. Tontisirin. Thonburi: P.I. Printing, 1992.

Winikoff, B. "Modification of Hospital Practices to Remove Obstacles to Successful Breastfeeding." Pp. 279–285 in *Programmes to Promote Breastfeeding*, edited by Dereck B. N. Jelliffe, and E. F. Patrice Jelliffe. Oxford: Oxford Medical Publications, 1987.

Winikoff, B, and E. Baer. "The Obstetrician's Opportunity: Translating 'Breast is Best' from Theory to Practice." *American Journal of Obstetrics & Gynecology* 138 (1980): 105–115.

Winikoff, B., S. Durongdej, B.J. "Infant Feeding in Bangkok, Thailand." Pp. 15–42 in *Feeding Infants in Four Societies: Causes and Consequences of Mothers' Choices*, edited by Beverley Winikoff, Mary A. Castle and Virginia H. Laukaran. New York: Greenwood Press, 1988.

Wongboonsin, K. *Population Policy and Programmes in Thailand: 1929–Present.* Publication No. 220/95. Bangkok: Institute of Population Studies, Chulalongkorn University, 1995.

Woollett, A., and A. Phoenix. "Psychological Views of Mothering." Pp. 28–46 in *Motherhood: Meanings, Practices and Ideologies*, edited by Ann Phoenix, Anne Woollett and Eva Lloyd. London: Sage, 1991.

Woolridge, M. "Baby-Controlled Feeding: Biocultural Implications." Pp. 168–217 in *Breastfeeding: Biocultural Perspectives*, edited by Patricia Stuart-Macadam and Katherine A. Dettwyler. New York: Aldine De Gruyer, 1995.

World Facts Index. *Chiang Mai*, 2004. http://worldfacts.us/Thailand-Chiang-Mai.htm. (Accessed December 20, 2004).

World Health Organization. *Breastfeeding: The Technical Basis and Recommendations for Action.* Geneva: WHO, 1993.

World Health Organization. *Not Enough Milk.* Geneva: Division of Diarrhoeal and Acute Respiratory Disease Control, WHO, 1996.

World Health Organization. *Infant and Young Child Nutrition: Global Strategy on Infant and Young Child Feeding.* Fifty-fifth World Health Assembly, Geneva: WHO, 2002.

Wright A.L., C. Clark, and M. Bauer. "Maternal Employment and Infant Feeding Practices among the Navajo." *Medical Anthropology Quarterly* 7 (1993): 260–280.

Wu, W-L. "Cesarean Delivery in Shantou, China: A Retrospective Analysis of 1922 Women." *Birth* 27(2) (2000): 86–90.

Yelland, J., R. Small, J. Lumley, P. Liamputtong Rice, V. Cotronei, and R. Warren. "Support, Sensitivity, Satisfaction: Vietnamese, Turkish and Filipino Women's Experience of the Postnatal Stay." *Midwifery* 14(3) (1998): 144–154.

Yimyam, S. *Breastfeeding Experiences Among Employed Women in Chiang Mai: Complexities of Combining Women's Roles.* Unpublished doctoral thesis, Key Centre for Women's Health in Society, The University of Melbourne, Melbourne, Australia, 1997.

Yimyam, S., and M. Morrow. "Breastfeeding Practices Among Employed Thai Women in Chiang Mai." *Journal of Human Lactation* 15(3) (1999): 225–232.

Yimyam, S., and M. Morrow. "Maternal Labor, Breast-Feeding, and Infant Health." Pp. 105–135 in *Global Inequalities at Work: Work's Impact on the Health of Individuals, Families, and Societies*, edited by Jody Heymann. New York: Oxford University Press, 2003.

Yimyam, S., M. Morrow, and W. Srisuphan. "Role Conflict and Rapid Socio-Economic Change: Breastfeeding among Employed Women in Thailand." *Social Science & Medicine* 49 (1999): 957–965.

Yip, P.S.F., J. Lee, and Y.B. Cheung. "The Influence of the Chinese Zodiac on Fertility in Hong Kong SAR." *Social Science & Medicine* 55 (2002): 1803–1812.

Young, E. *The Kingdom of the Yellow Robe*, 3rd edition. London: Archibald Constable, 1907.

Zadoroznyj, M. "Social Class, Social Selves and Social Control in Childbirth." *Sociology of Health & Illness* 21(3) (1999): 267–289.

Zanetta, G., A. Tampieri, I. Currado, A. Regalia, A. Nespoli, F. Fei, C. Colombo, and S. Bottino. "Changes in Cesarean Delivery in an Italian University Hospital, 1982–1996: A Comparison with the National Trend." *Birth* 26(3) (1999): 144–148.

Zeitlyn, S., and R. Rowshan. "Privileged Knowledge and Mother's 'Perceptions': The Case of Breast-Feeding and Insufficient Milk in Bangladesh." *Medical Anthropology Quarterly* 11(1) (1997): 56–68.

Index

Mayan mother/culture, 162
Medical anthropologist, 27
Medical dominance, 24, 29, 47, 49, 73, 94, 95, 105, 107, 181
Medical professional, and advice and recommendation, 30, 35, 38–40, 45, 46, 47, 48, 64–65, 68–69, 74, 81, 106, 148–152; and authoritative knowledge, 27–50, 148–152; and authority, 23, 24, 29, 33, 46, 148–152; and control over women's body, 30, 70, 73, 86, 105; and esoteric knowledge, 16, 86, 87; and fiduciary ethic, 68; and financial incentive, 69; and medical knowledge, 16, 24, 30, 32, 33, 34, 45, 46, 47, 68–69, 76, 86; and sanction, 30; and status, 24, 107; and trust in medical profession by women, 24, 30, 31, 35, 37, 46, 64–65, 68–69, 74, 84, 87, 148–152; power and knowledge, 28, 46, 47, 48, 49
Medical technology, 16, 23; and childbirth, 51–71, 52, 55, 56, 57, 59, 66, 67–69, 71, 73, 74, 76, 77; and empowerment, 55, 56, 67–69; and perception of risk, 55–56, 59, 69–71; and pregnancy, 36–37, 47; and resistance, 55, 67; and the well-being of infant, 58–59, 68–69; artificial rupture of membrane, 67; forceps, 59, 67, 85; induction, 59, 61; vacuum suction, 59, 60, 67, 84, 85
Middle-class women, 1, 17–18, 23, 24, 30; and caesarean birth, 51–71; and childbirth experience, 51–71, 73–91; and choice and control, 35, 48, 49, 53–55, 56, 66–67, 68, 74–75; and choice of birthing care, 57–58, 66–69; and financial resource, 23, 66; and infant care and childrearing, 155–179; and infant feeding practice, 127–154; and motherhood, 109–126; and postpartum belief and practice,

93–108; and pregnancy, 27–50; and rejection of medical control, 55–56, 67; empowerment, 55, 56, 66, 68, 69
Midwife, 13, 16, 34, 49, 84, 85, 142
Million Rice Fields Kingdom, 19
Ministry of Interior Affairs, 12
Ministry of Public Health, 11, 12
Miscarriage, 7, 33, 37, 39, 40, 46, 161
Modern medicine, 16, 95, 107
Modernity/modernization, 10, 11, 24, 44–45, 52, 56, 67, 70, 74, 86, 89, 93, 94, 95, 103–105, 107, 131, 135, 157, 158, 167
Mor boran, 14, (see *ya phaen boran*)
Mor muang, 100, 175 (see traditional healer)
Mor tamyae, 14 (see *mae jang* and traditional birth attendance)
Moral career, 111–112, 124
Moral women, 3
Motherhood, 1, 2, 6; and appreciation of one's own mother, 115–117, 125; and blame, 30, 68–69, 158; and emotional aspect, 110, 155–156, 181; and ethics of care, 111–112, 123; and expectation, 109, 124; and happiness and pride, 112–113, 123; and health, 25, 111, 117–120, 125–126; and identity, 110, 111–112, 147, 154, 158; and infant care, 155–179; and infant feeding, 127–154; and joy, 110, 113, 123; and maturity, 114–115, 124; and moral identity, 3, 4, 147, 154, 158, 158–159; and mothering role, 112, 155, 182; and "other" mother, 125; and relationship with husband and family member, 111, 120–122; and responsibility, 30, 111–112, 114–115, 123, 124, 156–159, 181; and reward, 109; and security in old age, 112–113, 179; and self-perception as mother, 111–112; and self-sacrifice and endless concern, 113–114, 124, 139; and social class, 109–126, 181–182;

About the Author

ﬡ

Pranee Liamputtong is Personal Chair in Public Health at the School of Public Health, La Trobe University, Melbourne, Australia. Pranee was born in Thailand and is now living in Australia. She has two daughters. Pranee has previously taught in the School of Sociology and Anthropology and worked as a public health research fellow at the Centre for the Study of Mothers' and Children's Health, La Trobe University. Pranee has her particular interests on issues related to cultural and social influences on childbearing, childrearing, and women's reproductive and sexual health. She has published several books and a large number of papers in these areas.

Her recent books include: *Asian Mothers, Western Birth* (new edition of *Asian Mothers, Australian Birth*, 1999); *Living in a New Country: Understanding Migrants' Health* (editor, 1999); *Hmong Women and Reproduction* (2000); *Coming of Age in South and Southeast Asia: Youth, Courtship and Sexuality* (with Lenore Manderson, 2002); and *Health, Social Change and Communities* (with Heather Gardner, 2003). Her most recent books include: *Reproduction, Childbearing and Motherhood: A Cross-Cultural Perspective*, and *Childrearing and Infant Care: A Cross-Cultural Perspective* (2007). She is in the process of completing *Population Health and Health Promotion: Principles and Process* (with Sansnee Jirojwong).

Her first research method book is titled *Qualitative Research Methods: A Health Focus* (with Douglas Ezzy, 1999, reprinted in 2000, 2001, 2003, 2004); and the second edition of this book is titled *Qualitative Research Methods* (2005). Her recent books include: *Health Research in Cyberspace: Methodological, Practical and Personal Issues* (2006), and *Researching the Vulnerable: A Guide to Sensitive Research Methods* (2006). She is completing a book on *Knowing Differently: An Introduction to Experiential and Art-Based Research Methods* (with Jean Rumbold). She is now working on *Doing Cross-Cultural Research: Methodological and Ethical Perspectives*, and *Undertaking Sensitive Research: Managing Boundaries, Emotions and Risk* (with Virginia Dickson-Swift and Erica James).